AF342174

Lung Oscillometry

Testing and Interpretation

Lung Oscillometry
Testing and Interpretation

Editor

Thomas Vadakkan

MD, DRCP (UK), Dip Boston, FCCS

Professor and DM Faculty

Department of Pulmonary Medicine

Amala Institute of Medical Sciences, Thrissur

Co-Editor

Nishanth PS

MD, FSM (ISDA), FCCS

DM Pulmonary Medicine and Critical Care Resident

Amala Institute of Medical Sciences, Thrissur

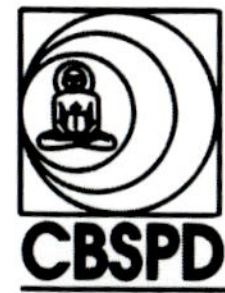

CBS Publishers & Distributors Pvt Ltd

New Delhi • Bengaluru • Chennai • Kochi • Kolkata • Lucknow • Mumbai
Hyderabad • Jharkhand • Nagpur • Patna • Pune • Uttarakhand

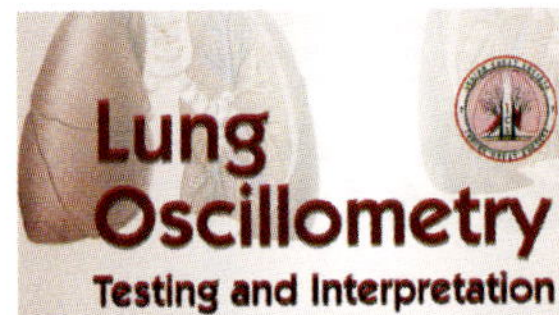

ISBN: 978-93-5466-966-8

Copyright © Editors and Publisher

First Edition: 2025

Published by Satish Kumar Jain and produced by Varun Jain for

CBS Publishers & Distributors Pvt Ltd

4819/XI Prahlad Street, 24 Ansari Road, Daryaganj, New Delhi 110 002, India
Ph: 011-23289259, 23266838

Website: www.cbspd.com
e-mail: delhi@cbspd.com

Corporate Office: 204 FIE, Industrial Area, Patparganj, Delhi 110 092, India
Ph: 011-49344934   Fax: 011-49344935   e-mail: publishing@cbspd.com; publicity@cbspd.com

Branches

- **Bengaluru:** Seema House 2975, 17th Cross, K.R. Road, Banasankari 2nd Stage, Bengaluru 560 070, Karnataka, India
  Ph: +91-80-26771678/79   Fax: +91-80-26771680   e-mail: bangalore@cbspd.com

- **Chennai:** 18/8B, Subbarayan Street, Shenoy Nagar, Chennai 600 030, Tamil Nadu, India
  Ph: +91-44-42032115, 26681266   e-mail: chennai@cbspd.com

- **Kochi:** 42/1325, 1326, Power House Road, Opposite KSEB, Power House, Ernakulum 682 018, Kochi, Kerala, India
  Ph: +91-484-4059061–65   Fax: +91-484-4059065   e-mail: kochi@cbspd.com

- **Kolkata:** 147, Hind Ceramics Compound, 1st Floor, Nilgunj Road, Belghoria, Kolkata 700 056, West Bengal, India
  Ph: +91-33-25330055/56   e-mail: kolkata@cbspd.com

- **Lucknow:** Basement, Khushuma Complex, 7 Meerabai Marg (behind Jawahar Bhawan), Lucknow 226 001, UP, India
  Ph: +91-522-4000032   e-mail: tiwari.lucknow@cbspd.com

- **Mumbai:** PWD Shed, Gala No. 25/26, Ramchandra Bhatt Marg, Next JJ Hospital Gate No. 2, Opp. Union Bank of India, Noorbaug, Mumbai 400 009, Maharashtra, India
  Ph: +91-22-66661880/89   e-mail: mumbai@cbspd.com

Representatives

• **Hyderabad**	0-9885175004	• **Jharkhand**	0-9811541605	• **Nagpur**	0-8692091830
• **Patna**	0-9334159340	• **Pune**	0-9664372571	• **Uttarakhand**	0-9716462459

Printed in Magic International Pvt. Ltd., Greater Noida, UP, India

to

Our families and mentors

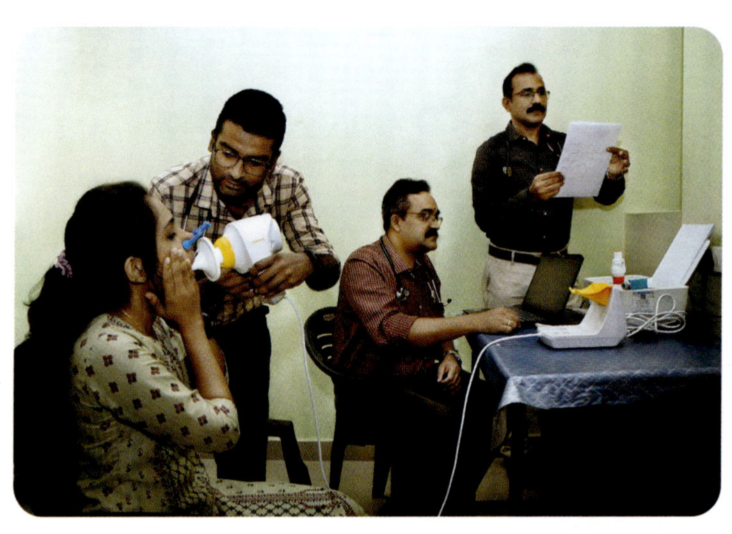

List of Contributors

Akhil Paul MD, DNB, EDARM, MRCP_SCE, IPGDFM, FCCP, FAPSR
Head
Department of Pulmonary Medicine
MOSC Medical Mission Hospital
Thrissur

Charu Singh
Respiratory Therapist (SIU)
Clinical Research and Customer Support
THORASYS Thoracic Medical Systems Inc
Montreal, Canada

Daksh Sharma MD, FCCS
DM Pulmonary Medicine and Critical Care Resident
Amala Institute of Medical Sciences
Thrissur

EV Krishnakumar MD, DTCD
Professor
Department of Respiratory Medicine
Amala Institute of Medical Sciences
Thrissur

Lennart KA Lundblad PhD
Director
Department of Clinical Science
THORASYS Thoracic Medical Systems Inc
Associate Professor
McGill University, Montreal
Canada

Manju Rajaram MD
Professor and Ex-Head
Department of Pulmonary Medicine
JIPMER, Puducherry

Muniza Bai MD, DNB, EDARM
DM Pulmonary Medicine and Critical Care Resident
AIIMS, New Delhi

Nishanth PS MD, FSM (ISDA), FCCS
DM Pulmonary Medicine and Critical Care Resident
Amala Institute of Medical Sciences
Thrissur

R Venkateswara Babu MD (TB & RD)
Professor and Head
Department of Respiratory Medicine
IGMCRI, Puducherry

Thomas Vadakkan MD, DRCP (UK), Dip Boston, FCCS
Professor and DM Faculty
Department of Pulmonary Medicine
Amala Institute of Medical Sciences
Thrissur

Venugopal J MD, DNB, EDARM, FCCP
Consultant
Interventional Pulmonologist
KMCH, Coimbatore

Foreword

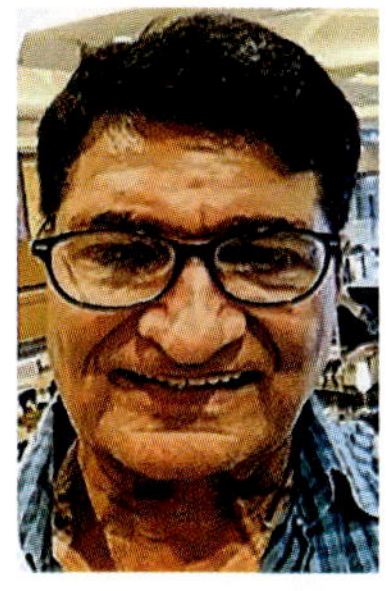

I am very pleased to write the Foreword for book written by one of my students who graduated from JIPMER, an institution of excellence. Dr Thomas Vadakkan completed his postgraduate training in pulmonary medicine at JIPMER and is currently a professor in the Department of Pulmonary Medicine at the Amala Institute of Medical Sciences in Thrissur. I, myself being an editor of the Indian Journal of Tuberculosis, and I sit down everyday to write comments and notes about various manuscripts submitted. I am familiar with this task, but when your own student asks for a Foreword for his book, it seems a bit challenging.

This book has been authored by Dr Thomas Vadakkan, with contributions from multiple authors, for advancement of knowledge in oscillometry. Oscillometry tool is now being used in both the private and government sectors, and it seems that with time and further improvements in the available equipment, it may replace spirometry.

Writing and editing a book is a significant responsibility, especially when it is the first of its kind to be written in India. I congratulate Dr Thomas Vadakkan and Co-Editor, Dr Nishanth PS (who completed his postgraduate training in Amritsar), for creating such an excellent book. This book is a collaborative effort by different authors, not only focusing on lung function but also delving into the physics underlying oscillometry practice. Restrictive and obstructive diseases have traditionally been diagnosed through spirometry, which requires coordination of respiratory muscles, and the chapter clearly shows that oscillometry simplifies this process especially in elderly and children by using simple tidal breathing for approximately 30 seconds.

The chapters written are of high quality, providing an excellent framework for lung function assessment with oscillometry. Creating nomograms for the elderly and children in the Indian context has been well identified.

I believe that this book will be very useful for postgraduate students and teachers in medical colleges and deserves a place in the library of each medical college.

Once again, I congratulate Dr Thomas Vadakkan and Dr Nishanth PS (Co-Editor) for their efforts in writing a book that will serve as a reference in the times to come.

Best Wishes!

VK Arora
MD, DCD, CTC & E (Japan), FNCCP, FIMSA, FCAM, FGSI
Chairman
Tuberculosis Association of India

Foreword

It is with great pleasure that I introduce you this comprehensive book on lung oscillometry, a multidimensional exploration authored by experts from subject. The book covers history, physics, physiology, and clinical practice related to lung oscillometry. This collaborative effort represents a remarkable journey through the intricate landscape of lung function assessment, leveraging the power of oscillometry as a pivotal tool in understanding respiratory health and disease.

The history of medical advancement is marked by seminal moments where pioneering minds intersected across disciplines, propelling our understanding forward. In a world grappling with the complexities of respiratory conditions, this book serves as a beacon of such interdisciplinary brilliance. Comprising contributions from luminaries in their respective domains, this book bridges historical insight with modern breakthroughs, unifying the past and present in a cohesive narrative.

The opening chapters delve into the historical evolution of lung function assessment, tracing its origins and the milestones that paved the way for oscillometry's integration in clinical practice. As we move deeper into the text, the physics underlying lung oscillometry come to the forefront. The authors illuminate the intricate principles that govern the interaction between respiratory systems and oscillatory signals, providing readers with a solid foundation to understand the method's mechanics.

Physiology takes centre stage as we transition into the heart of the book. With a meticulous analysis of the oscillometric parameters, the authors unlock the potential of this technique to elucidate the underlying mechanisms of normal and pathological respiratory function. 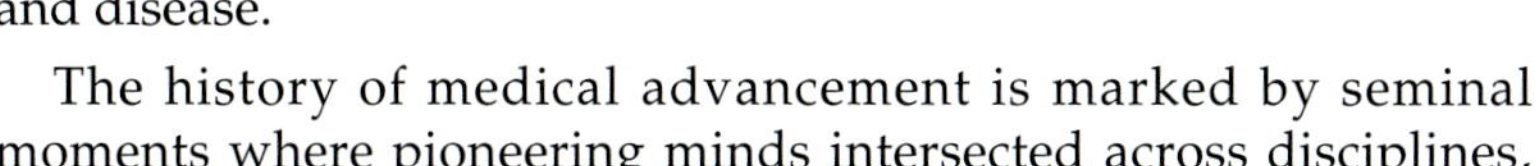 Through insightful case studies and real-world applications, readers gain invaluable insights into the role of oscillometry in diagnosing and monitoring a spectrum of lung conditions. 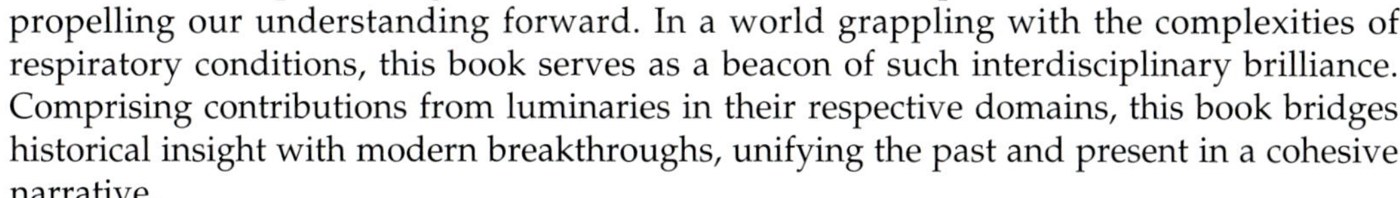

No exploration of a medical technique is complete without addressing potential pitfalls and troubleshooting strategies. The authors deftly guide us through the challenges that may arise in the application of oscillometry, offering pragmatic solutions grounded in their extensive clinical experience. A dedicated section comparing oscillometry to spirometry underscores the unique advantages and complementary roles these techniques play in clinical evaluation.

The book then pivots towards a comprehensive analysis of oscillometry's impact in the context of obstructive and restrictive lung diseases. Through an astute integration of physiology, pathology, and clinical observation, the authors offer readers a panoramic view of how oscillometry contributes to unravelling the complex tapestry of respiratory disorders.

As we march forward, the authors bring us face-to-face with the cutting-edge developments in oscillometry. This is a testament to the dynamism of medical science, as emerging technologies reshape the landscape of lung function assessment. The authors reveal how recent advances have pushed the boundaries of our understanding, allowing clinicians and researchers to explore new dimensions of respiratory health.

The journey culminates in a section dedicated to nomograms, presenting readers with a visual representation of normative data for various populations. This compendium of knowledge is an invaluable reference point, enabling healthcare professionals to interpret oscillometric data with precision and contextual accuracy.

In closing, this textbook is an embodiment of collective wisdom, a testament to the transformative potential that emerges when diverse minds converge to dissect a critical facet of medical science. Whether you are a seasoned clinician, an aspiring researcher, or simply curious about the intricate dance of respiratory physiology, this book promises to be an illuminating companion on your journey.

Mohankumar Thekkinkattil

MD, DPPR, FCCP, FAARC, FAPSR,

President-Elect National College of Chest Physicians

Past President of 1. Indian Chest Society, 2. Indian Association of Bronchology,

3. Academy of Pulmonary and Critical Care Medicine, 4. Coimbatore Respiratory Society

Past Chair/Secretary: Clinical Problems ERS

Past International Governor ACCP, AARC

Senior Consultant Pulmonologist and Head

One Care Medical Centre, Coimbatore, India

Foreword

In the realm of modern medicine, knowledge is our compass, and innovation our guiding star. As we navigate the uncharted waters of pulmonary diagnostics, the role of oscillometry shines brightly as a beacon of progress. This book, a testament to the tireless efforts of dedicated experts, unveils the intricacies of oscillometry and its pivotal role in the ever-evolving landscape of pulmonary function testing. Spirometry has its own limitations in assessing pulmonary function. Oscillometry being more objective and offers a new horizon for clinicians, researchers, and students alike. This book not only demystifies the intricacies of oscillometry but also provides valuable insights into its applications across various pulmonary conditions.

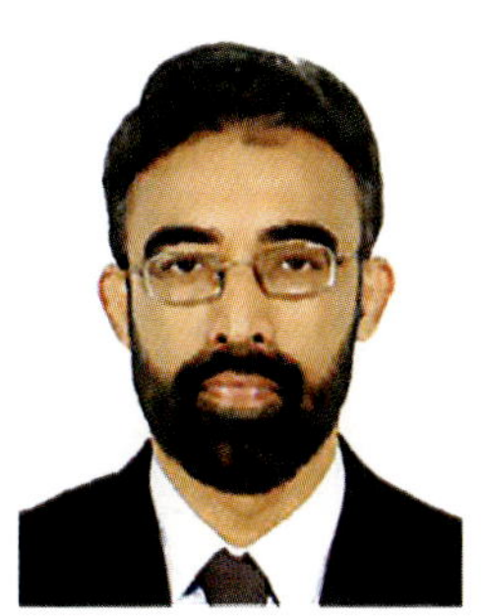

Within these pages, readers will embark on a journey through the principles, techniques, and applications of oscillometry. Each chapter is a testament to the dedication and passion of the authors. As we delve into the depths of this field, we uncover its potential to enhance the accuracy of pulmonary assessments, optimize patient care, and contribute to the advancement of respiratory medicine. In an age where healthcare is more data-driven than ever before, understanding oscillometry is not just a choice; it is a necessity. This book serves as a comprehensive guide, a source of inspiration, and a resource for those who seek to embrace the future of pulmonary diagnostics. It is my privilege to introduce you to this invaluable resource, which I am confident will not only broaden your horizons but also deepen your appreciation for the vital role oscillometry plays in the pursuit of healthier lives.

May your exploration of these pages be enlightening and may your application of oscillometry lead to improved patient outcomes and a brighter future for respiratory healthcare.

Davis Paul
Professor and Head, Department of Respiratory Medicine
Amala Institute of Medical Sciences
Thrissur
President of APCCM

Preface

The study of physiology of lungs traditionally relies upon spirometry, which presents challenges when applied to both elderly individuals and the pediatric population. Lung oscillometry has emerged as a promising alternative, though it is not a complete replacement for spirometry within the current framework of clinical practice. Notably, the availability of textbooks, handbooks, and literature about lung oscillometry remains limited. Consequently, the present endeavour seeks to compile and consolidate contemporary knowledge and data pertaining to lung oscillometry, providing a valuable resource for practising chest physicians, pediatricians, and budding pulmonologists.

This compilation carries diverse facets of lung oscillometry, encompassing foundational principles, physiology, methodological techniques, and nuanced interpretation. Moreover, to enhance the educational value of this resource, a selection of practice questions, complete with answers and explanations, are included at the end of this book. It is worth noting that nomogram of lung oscillometry still remains a grey area necessitating expansive research to establish nomogram for each population.

I extend profound gratitude to all the esteemed authors who diligently contributed to the timely completion of this comprehensive work. A special note of thanks to my DM Residents, Dr Nishanth PS and Dr Daksh Sharma, whose efforts have transformed this textbook into a reality. It is with immense pleasure that I thank the organizers of NAPCON 2023 Hyderabad for offering us the opportunity to write this authoritative text about lung oscillometry.

Thomas Vadakkan

Contents

Abbreviations

1. FEV_1: Forced expiratory volume in 1 second

2. FVC: Forced vital capacity

3. PEFR: Peak expiratory flow rate

4. $FEF_{25-75\%}$: Forced expiratory flow between 25–75% of FVC

5. Z_{rs}: Respiratory impedance

6. R_{rs}: Respiratory resistance

7. X_{rs}: Respiratory reactance

8. F_{res}: Resonant frequency

9. A_x: Reactance area

10. R_5: Respiratory resistance at 5 Hz

11. X_5: Respiratory reactance at 5 Hz

History of Impulse Oscillometry

• Venugopal J

Spirometry, the most commonly performed pulmonary function test is the standard of care in the diagnosis of obstructive airway disease. Spirometry helps to assess the severity of obstruction, also helps to assess the response to treatment. However, the forceful inhalational and exhalational maneuvers in spirometry make this test a little complex especially in paediatric and geriatric population.[1] In this subset of population, impulse oscillometry plays an important role in the diagnostic and prognostic workup.

Sound waves are used in impulse oscillometry, a non-invasive technique for measuring respiratory mechanics. It is based on the forced oscillation technique (FOT) concept, which Dubios et al originally explained in 1956.[2] As a pioneer in the field of oscillometry, Authur Dubois proposed the technique of analyzing the mechanical characteristics of the airways during tidal breathing when high-frequency oscillating pressure was applied (Fig. 1.1). They used a special equipment that creates sinusoidal sound waves, which are transmitted to the airways during normal breathing.[3] In 1968, Grimby and associates proposed that oscillation frequencies play a major factor in determining the airway resistance in patients with obstructive lung disorders (Fig. 1.1).[4]

It was Arthur Dubois who first proposed a novel technique for estimating a person's lung capacity in a sealed chamber by monitoring variations in pressure at the mouth (Fig. 1.2). After this creation, body plethysmography became popular in pulmonology. However, for many years oscillometry technique was not widely used by the physicians. This is because it involves sophisticated physics. Using a rapid Fourier transform, oscillometry converts signals from the time domain to the frequency domain. It then produces imaginary or negative numbers for reactance values. Many doctors found it difficult because of the advanced physics involved, and the second problem was primarily technological.[5]

In 1976 Michealson created a modified oscillometry technique: Impulse oscillometry was born.[6] Impulse oscillometry delivers regular square waves of pressure 5 times per second, which has the advantage of producing larger sample during measurement and transmitting a continuous frequency spectrum that can provide a more detailed analysis of respiratory mechanics.

Because the pioneers constructed their own oscillometric system and data analysis was done manually, the original studies were time-consuming.[5,6] The discovery of advanced calculations, along with the development of pressure transducers that accurately evaluate pressure changes at high frequency, enabled the development of a commercial system. Later this IOS was commercialized by Jaeger.

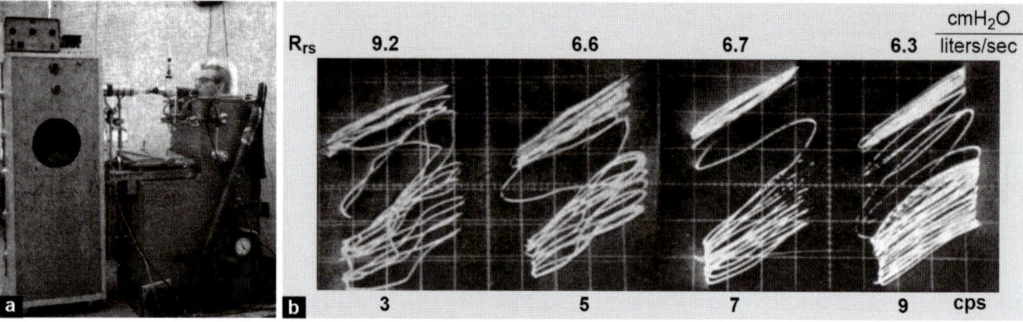

Fig. 1.1: Dubois oscillometry machine

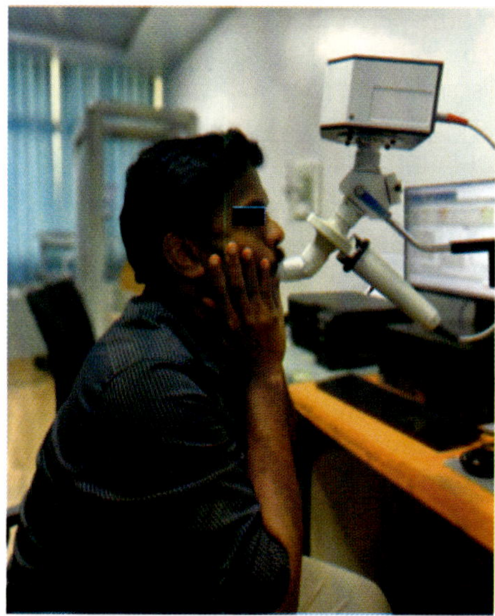

Fig. 1.2: Newer version of oscillometry machine

REFERENCES

1. Gupta N, Sachdev A, Gupta D, Gupta S. Oscillometry–The future of estimating pulmonary functions. Karnataka Paediatr J 2020;35(2):79–87.

2. Desiraju, Koundinya, Agrawal, Anurag. Impulse oscillometry: The state-of-art for lung function testing. Lung India 2016;33(4):410–16.

3. AB Dubois, AW Brody, DH Lewis, BF Burgess. Oscillation mechanics of lungs and chest in man. J. Appl. Physiol. 1956;8(6):587–94, https://doi.org/10.1152/ jappl.1956.8.6.587.

4. Michaelson ED, Grassman ED, Peters WR. Pulmonary mechanics by spectral analysis of forced random noise. J Clin Invest. 1975 Nov;56(5):1210–30. doi: 10.1172/JCI108198. PMID: 1184746; PMCID: PMC301985.

5. Calverley PMA, Farré R. Oscillometry: Old physiology with a bright future. Eur Respir J. 2020 Sep 10;56(3):2001815. doi: 10.1183/13993003.01815-2020. PMID: 32912925.

6. Grimby G, Takishima T, Graham W, et al. Frequency dependence of flow resistance in patients with obstructive lung disease. J Clin Invest 1968;47:1455–65. doi:10.1172/JCI105837.

Physics and Physiology of Oscillometry

• *Charu Singh* • *Lennart KA Lundblad*

Oscillometry measures lung impedance with exceptional sensitivity to alterations in respiratory mechanics.[1] It is particularly adept at detecting changes in the peripheral lung and small airways, areas not well assessed by conventional pulmonary function tests.[2]

Research on oscillometry is growing, with a rising focus on its clinical application due to increased interest and feasibility. Respiratory oscillometry assesses the mechanical characteristics of the respiratory system, including the upper and intrathoracic airways, lung tissue, and chest wall, through the introduction of small pressure or flow oscillations (input or forcing signal) during quiet tidal breathing, typically applied at the mouth.

While the fundamental principles of oscillometry measurement remain consistent across all devices, variations in hardware, data acquisition, signal processing, and breathing protocols can result in discrepancies in impedance measurements. Additionally, it is important to note that oscillometry represents a distinct measurement from traditional lung function assessments, such as spirometry and lung volumes. This section delves into the underlying physics of oscillometry, exploring concepts like impedance, resistive and reactive components, and the resonance phenomenon.[3,4]

Typically, this method is employed to passively assess the mechanical characteristics of the respiratory system, eliminating the need for active maneuvers like forced expiration. Oscillations can be introduced during spontaneous tidal breathing or respiratory support ventilation, proving highly valuable in various clinical scenarios not covered by routine tests, especially in young children and during mechanical ventilation. In oscillometry testing, a stimulus is applied to the respiratory system at the mouth. The input signal can be either pressure or flow oscillation, and the corresponding response (in terms of flow or pressure, respectively) is measured. The ratio of oscillatory pressure to oscillatory flow resulting from this stimulus is utilized to calculate input impedance, offering a comprehensive representation of the overall mechanical properties of the respiratory system.

STIMULATION TERMINOLOGY

There is considerable ambiguity in the terminology related to oscillometry, with terms such as "FOT" for "forced oscillation technique" and "IOS" or "iOS" for "impulse oscillometry" often used interchangeably. While both methods involve oscillation mechanics, they employ different stimuli to achieve a common objective: Vibrating an air column from the mouth to the alveolus and the surrounding tissue to assess the mechanical properties of the respiratory system—specifically, impedance and its three components: Resistance, elastance, and inertance.

The term "forced" in FOT pertains to the compelling nature of sine waves on the respiratory system. These waves control approximately 10 cc volume oscillations, assuming a healthy subject, during both the upward and downward phases of the volume change. Unlike FEV_1, the term "forced" is unrelated to the subject's maneuver, as they only need to breathe quietly for typically 16–30 seconds.

In contrast, IOS utilizes an impulse or square wave to vibrate the air column from the mouth to the alveolus. Some devices deliver only sine waves, others only impulses, and some offer the capability to use either. To alleviate confusion associated with terms like "forced," the author recommends using the term "oscillometry" or "OSC," which accurately encompasses all devices and stimulation modes while avoiding potential confusion.

IMPEDANCE OF THE RESPIRATORY SYSTEM

In the realm of oscillometry, impedance pertains to the resistance encountered by the respiratory system against the flow of oscillatory pressure signals. It is expressed as the ratio of oscillatory pressure to oscillatory flow and can be defined by the following equation:

$$Z(\omega) = Q(\omega)/P(\omega)$$

where $Z(\omega)$ is the impedance, $P(\omega)$ is the oscillatory pressure, and $Q(\omega)$ is the oscillatory flow. Impedance can be further divided into two main components: Resistive and reactive.

Resistive Component

The resistive component of impedance is primarily influenced by the frictional losses occurring within the airways as air flows through them. This is associated with the viscosity of the air and the geometry of the airways. In oscillometry, the resistive component is characterized by the frequency-independent resistance (R).

Mathematically, the relationship between pressure and flow for the resistive component can be expressed as:

$$P(\omega) = R{\cdot}Q(\omega)$$

Reactive Component

The reactive component of impedance arises due to the elastic properties of the lung tissues and airways. It is influenced by factors such as lung compliance and inertia. The reactive component is characterized by the frequency-dependent reactance (X).
The relationship between pressure and flow for the reactive component can be expressed as:

$$P(\omega) = X{\cdot}i{\cdot}\omega{\cdot}Q(\omega)$$

where i is the imaginary unit, and is the angular frequency of the oscillation.

RESONANCE PHENOMENON

A crucial aspect of oscillometry is the resonance phenomenon. In a healthy respiratory system, there exists a resonant frequency (F_{res}) at which the impedance is minimized. This frequency corresponds to the point where the reactive component is maximally negative, canceling out the positive resistive component. At this resonant frequency, energy transfer between the oscillatory pressure signal and the oscillatory flow signal is most efficient.[5–7]

The Physiology and Performance of Oscillometry

Oscillometry quantifies the mechanical impedance of the respiratory system (Z_{rs}), which encompasses the resistive and reactive forces that must be surmounted to propel an oscillating flow signal into the respiratory system. These forces originate within the respiratory system due to:

1. Resistance to flow within the airways and tissues (R_{rs}),
2. Elastance (stiffness) exhibited by the lung parenchyma and chest wall in response to volume changes (incorporated in reactance, X_{rs}), and
3. Inertance resulting from the acceleration of gas in the airways (I_{rs}).

Z_{rs} is typically reported as an average across the entire breathing cycle (both inspiration and expiration) from a single frequency or over the frequency range of 5–40 Hz. Additionally, it has been separately documented during the inspiratory and expiratory phases.

Impedance

Respiratory impedance encompasses all the opposing forces to the generated impulse. The impedance measured at a specific frequency is the ratio of the pressure difference to the changes in flow at that frequency. The variation in impedance depends on the region where the pressure is measured. For instance, the pressure difference at the mouth and in the alveoli provides the impedance of the airways, while the difference at the mouth and pleural pressures yields the total impedance of the lung. In oscillometry, the pressure measured at the mouth is compared to atmospheric pressure, which represents the pressure outside the chest wall.[8]

Respiratory system impedance reflects the cumulative forces associated with resistance, elastance, and inertance that need to be overcome for driving airflow into and out of the lung. Z_{rs} broadly characterizes the mechanical properties of the entire respiratory system, including the airway, parenchyma, and chest wall. Z_{rs} itself is not utilized in clinical practice. Instead, it is represented by its components, respiratory system resistance (R_{rs}) and reactance (X_{rs}), described as follows.

This is defined as the respiratory system Z_{rs} and comprises the in-phase (real) component, which is the resistive component (R_{rs}), and an out-of-phase (imaginary) component, which is a reactive component (X_{rs}). In simpler terms, Rrs can be regarded as energy dissipation, while X_{rs} represents energy storage (Fig. 2.1).

Resistance

The resistance derived from impedance encompasses the resistance associated with central airways, peripheral airways, lung tissue, and chest wall, although the latter two are typically negligible. Approximately 80% of the resistance is attributed to central airways, with only 20% contributed by small airways (those with a diameter of less than 2 mm) in adults.[22,23] This distribution is primarily due to the extensive total cross-sectional area of small airways. However, in children, the contribution of small airways is higher compared to adults. Normal resistance values are considered to fall within the range of 150% of predicted values. Resistance remains independent of frequency in healthy individuals.

In cases of central airway obstruction, the resistance increases at all frequencies, whereas in small airway obstruction, the resistance at lower frequencies increases while remaining unchanged at higher frequencies that do not reach the small airways. This frequency-

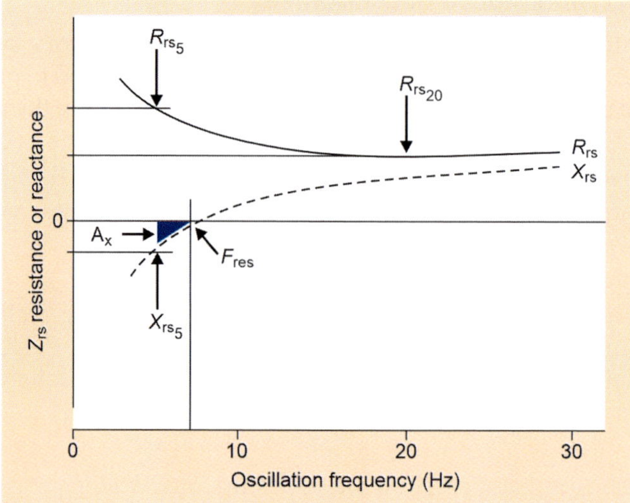

Fig. 2.1: Respiratory system resistance and reactance by impulse oscillometry

dependent pattern of resistance may be typical in children but signifies small airway obstruction in adults.

The resistance of the respiratory system mirrors frictional losses occurring both in gases as they traverse airways and in the tissues of the lung and chest wall as they undergo stretching and deformation. Individual frequencies of R_{rs} are denoted as R_{rs5}, R_{rs}, and so forth. Alterations in R_{rs} at frequencies above approximately 5 Hz are indicative of changes in airway resistance, specifically related to caliber, making them sensitive to airway constriction. Consequently, R_{rs} may increase in clinical scenarios such as bronchoconstriction, the presence of excessive mucus or mucus plugging, airway inflammation, and other conditions leading to airway narrowing or obstruction. Tissue resistance gains prominence as the frequency decreases below 5 Hz, becoming particularly significant at normal breathing frequencies (around 0.2 Hz) and lower.

Reactance

Reactance consists of two elements: The inertia of the air column to movement (inertance) and the capacitance of the lung, where capacitance reflects the lung's elasticity. The capacitance component of reactance is designated as negative, while inertance is positive. Unlike resistance, reactance varies with frequency. At low frequencies, where the elastic properties of the lungs are primarily peripheral, the capacitance component predominates, resulting in a negative total lung reactance. Conversely, at higher frequencies, the inertia of the air column in larger airways dominates, leading to a positive total reactance. Notably, elastance or capacitance in this context pertains to the lung's energy return properties, akin to electric circuits, rather than stiffness during inflation—a more intuitive definition for clinicians.

As a result, whether in fibrosis, emphysema, or small airway disease, reactance at lower frequencies changes in the same direction, becoming even more negative. Therefore, the alteration in reactance does not provide differentiation between obstructive or restrictive diseases.

The reactance of the respiratory system mirrors the elastance (E_{rs}) of the respiratory system, arising from the collective stiffness of the lung and chest wall tissues (below the resonance frequency, F_{res}, as described below), and the inertance (I_{rs}) of the respiratory system, stemming from the mass of gas in the central airways (above the resonance frequency). In lung diseases, X_{rs} tends to become "more negative," indicating an increase in respiratory system stiffness. X_{rs} is highly reliant on lung volume, and X_{rs5}, in particular, has been shown to be sensitive to airway closure, reflecting the communicating lung volume. Changes in X_{rs5} within a breath are valuable for detecting expiratory flow limitation. As of now, I_{rs} is not commonly employed as a clinical measure of lung disease, but it may undergo alterations in conditions that affect gas flow in the upper and central airways.

Resonant Frequency

The resonant frequency (F_{res}) is defined as the frequency at which the inertial properties of the airway and the capacitance of the lung periphery are balanced, resulting in a total reactance of zero. While we cannot attribute F_{res} to a specific mechanical property of the lungs, it serves to distinguish low frequencies where the capacitance component prevails from high frequencies where the inertial component takes precedence. The typical value of F_{res} in adults ranges from 7 to 12 Hz. In children, it is higher and tends to decrease with age. In lung diseases, both obstructive and restrictive, F_{res} is elevated above the normal range, as explained earlier when discussing the increased negativity of reactance at low frequencies in these conditions.

At the resonant frequency, E_{rs} and I_{rs} contribute equally and oppositely to impedance, resulting in a zero X_{rs}. E_{rs} has a predominant role in shaping X_{rs} as the frequency drops below F_{res}, while I_{rs} becomes increasingly dominant above F_{res}. The F_{res} for a healthy adult male is typically around 8 Hz but is usually higher in the presence of lung disease. In children, F_{res} generally surpasses 8 Hz and tends to decrease with age.

Area of Reactance

The area of reactance (A_x) entails the region beneath the reactance curve, extending from the lowest frequency to the resonant frequency (F_{res}). It corresponds to the space between the X-axis below zero and the reactance curve on the graph, encapsulating the entire area influenced by capacitance and mirroring the elastic characteristics of the lung. Similar to reactance and F_{res}, the A_x value elevates in the presence of any lung periphery disease. A_x serves as a consolidated measure that encapsulates the aforementioned parameters and has been demonstrated to correlate with resistance at lower frequencies.

Coherence

Coherence is another crucial parameter employed to assess the validity and quality of test results, indicating the reproducibility of impedance measurements. It is a numerical value falling between 0 and 1, with the ideal threshold being >0.8 at 5 Hz and >0.9 at 20 Hz for the measurement to be deemed valid. It is worth noting that these benchmarks are applicable to adults, and no standardized values have been established for children. Factors such as improper technique, irregular breathing, glottis closure, and swallowing can lead to a decrease in coherence.

Normal Healthy Subjects

The oscillogram and oscillometry parameters of a healthy adult subject commonly exhibit an almost flat resistance curve. Depending on age and height, R_5 values should be ≤2.0 to

3.0 cmH$_2$O.s/L. There is negligible frequency dependence, resulting in R$_{5-20}$ being close to 0, signifying the absence of small airway disease. The X$_5$ of the reactance curve is typically ≥2.0, and the F_{res} falls within the range of 8 to 15 Hz. A normal A$_x$ is <10 cm H$_2$O/L.

SUMMARY

Despite its existence for approximately six decades, oscillometry lacks the same level of standardization as spirometry. Consequently, there is a shortage of normative data for making comparisons. Currently, oscillometry has predominantly found application in clinical research. Although this represents a limitation, it has simultaneously provided the scientific community with a more comprehensive and nuanced comprehension of lung diseases compared to what could have been attained through spirometry alone.

The following oscillometry parameter definitions encompass all the necessary information for practitioners to effectively utilize oscillometry in a clinical setting:

1. **R$_5$:** Represents the resistance of the total respiratory system from the mouth to the body surface.

2. **Frequency dependence of resistance (R$_{5-19}$ or R$_{5-20}$):** Serves as a measure of heterogeneity among airway impedances due to time constant inequalities. For clinicians, it can be simplistically viewed as a sensitive measure of small airways disease. However, it may be influenced by upper airway and large airway shunting, and more frequently by conditions like morbid obesity.[9–14]

3. **X$_5$:** Primarily reflects the elastic or stiffness properties of the respiratory system and tends to worsen in obstructive lung disease.[15–18]

4. **F_{res}:** Denotes the point where the reactance curve intersects the 0-impedance line. At this juncture, capacitive and inertive forces cancel out, and impedance is solely attributable to resistance.[19–21]

5. **Reactance area (A$_x$):** Encompasses the region enclosed by the reactance curve, starting at X$_5$, F_{res}, and the y-axis 0 line. Recent findings suggest it serves as a reasonable estimate of ventilatory inhomogeneity.[22,23]

REFERENCES

1. Bates JH, Irvin CG, Farre R, Hanto s Z. Oscillation mechanics of the respiratory system. Comprehensive Physiology. 2011;1(3):1233–72.

2. Chang E, Vasileva A, Nohra C, Ryan CM, Chow CW, Wu JKY. Conducting Respiratory Oscillometry in an Outpatient Setting. J. Vis. Exp. (182), e63243, doi:10.3791/63243 (2022).

3. Lennart KA Lundblad, Salman Siddiqui, Ynuk Bossé and Ronald J. Dandurand (2021) Applications of oscillometry in clinical research and practice, Canadian Journal of Respiratory, Critical Care, and Sleep Medicine, 5:1, 54–68, DOI: 10.1080/24745332.2019.1649607.

4. Bates JH, Irvin CG, Farre R, Hantos Z. Oscillometry for lung function assessment in mice: theoretical and practical considerations. Journal of Applied Physiology. 2004;97(2):683–91.

5. Goldman MD, Saadeh C, Ross D. Clinical applications of forced oscillation to assess peripheral airway function. Respiratory Physiology and Neurobiology. 2005;148(1–2):179–94.

6. King GG, Bates JH. Using oscillometry to assess airway obstruction and as a guide to treatment. European Respiratory Journal. 2009;33(4):981–90.

7. Oostveen E, MacLeod D, Lorino H, et al. The forced oscillation technique in clinical practice: methodology, recommendations and future developments. European Respiratory Journal. 2003;22(6):1026–41.

8. Desiraju K, Agrawal A. Impulse oscillometry: The state-of-art for lung function testing. Lung India 2016;33:410–6.

9. Foy BH, Soares M, Bordas R, et al. Lung computational models and the role of the small airways in asthma. *Am J Respir Crit Care Med*. 2019. doi:10.1164/rccm.201812-2322OC.

10. Kaczka DW, Lutchen KR, Hantos Z. Emergent behavior of regional heterogeneity in the lung and its effects on respiratory impedance. *J Appl Physiol*. 2011;110:1473–81. doi:10.1152/japplphysiol.01287.2010

11. Desager KN, Cauberghs M, Naudts J, et al. Influence of upper airway shunt on total respiratory impedance in infants. *J Appl Physiol*. 1999;87:902–09. doi:10.1152/jappl.1999.87.3.902.72.

12. Bates JH, Allen GB. The estimation of lung mechanics parameters in the presence of pathology: a theoretical analysis. Ann Biomed Eng. 2006;34:384–92. doi:10.1007/s10439-005-9056-6.73.

13. Bhatawadekar SA, Leary D, Maksym GN. Modelling resistance and reactance with heterogeneous airway narrowing in mild to severe asthma. Can J Physiol Pharmacol. 2015;93:207–14. doi:10.1139/cjpp-2014-0436.74.

14. Cauberghs M, Van De Woestijne KP. Effect of upper airway shunt and series properties on respiratory impedance measurements. J Appl Physiol. 1989;66:2274–79. doi:10.1152/jappl.1989.66.5.2274.75.

15. Albuquerque CG, de Andrade FMD, de Rocha MA, de A, et al. Determining respiratory system resistance and reactance by impulse oscillometry in obese individuals. J Bras Pneumol. 2015;41:422–26. doi:10.1590/S1806-37132015000004517.

16. Naglaa BA, Kamal E. Role of IOS in evaluation of patients with interstitial lung diseases. Egypt J Chest Dis Tuberc. 2016;65:791–95. doi:10.1016/j.ejcdt.2016.05.002.

17. Dandurand R, Dandurand M, Estepar R, et al. Oscillometry incommunity practice ild is characterized by abnormal reactance but normal resistance. Quart J Med. 2016;109:S50. doi:10.1093/qjmed/hcw127.019.32.

18. Schuessler T, Drapeau G, Maksym G. Temporal variations of oscillometric reactance in COPD and ILD. *Eur Respir J*. 2015;46:PA514.

19. Eddy RL, Westcott A, Maksym GN, et al. Oscillometry and pulmonary magnetic resonance imaging in asthma and COPD. Physiol Rep. 2019;7:e13955. doi:10.14814/phy2.13955.

20. Kaminsky DA, Simpson SJ, Berger KI, et al. Clinical significance and applications of oscillometry. Eur Respir Rev 2022;31:210208 [DOI: 10.1183/16000617.0208-2021].

21. Li Q, Yi Q, Tang L, et al. Influence of ultrafine particles exposure on asthma exacerbation in children: a meta-analysis. Curr Drug Targets. 2018;20(4):412–20. http://dx.doi.org/10.2174/1389450119666180829114252.

22. Hogg JC, Williams J, Richardson JB, Macklem PT, Thurlbeck WM. Age as a factor in the distribution of lower-airway conductance and in the pathologic anatomy of obstructive lung disease. *N Engl J Med* 1970;282:1283–87.

23. Mead J. The lung's "quiet zone". *N Engl J Med* 1970;282:1318–19.

Performing and Troubleshooting Oscillometry

• Charu Singh • Lennart KA Lundblad

Respiratory oscillometry, an alternative approach to pulmonary function testing, is increasingly employed in both clinical and research settings to gather insights into lung mechanics. This technique involves three acceptable measurements of tidal breathing and can be carried out with minimal contraindications. Individuals, particularly young children or those with cognitive or physical limitations preventing spirometry, can typically undergo oscillometry successfully. Notably, respiratory oscillometry boasts advantages such as requiring minimal patient cooperation and displaying greater sensitivity in detecting changes in small airways compared to traditional pulmonary function tests. Commercial devices are now accessible, and recent publications include updated technical guidelines, standard operating protocols, and quality control/assurance guidelines. Additionally, reference values are readily available. Conducting oscillometry requires following a sequence of steps to guarantee precise and dependable measurements.

While the test is generally effort independent, the patient should be coached or trained by an experienced technician to guarantee a high quality test.

OSCILLOMETRY BACKGROUND

As noted earlier, the patient's involvement is minimal in oscillometry, as the signal for assessing lung mechanics is produced by a device delivering varying frequencies of pressure oscillations to the respiratory system. This frequency range typically spans from 5 Hz to around 40 Hz, and it is preferable for these frequencies to be non-harmonic prime frequencies to prevent harmonic interference. The oscillations in volume produce flow and pressure with identical frequency content, and through signal processing, dividing pressure by flow yields the impedance.

Preparation and Screening Before the Test

1. Confirm that the patient is not currently experiencing any active or suspected transmissible respiratory infections, such as coronavirus or tuberculosis.
2. Verify that the patient has not undergone recent dental or facial surgeries, like tooth extractions, and can create a secure seal around the mouthpiece.
3. Ensure the patient is in a relaxed state, not wearing tightly fitted clothing, and refrains from tobacco use and vigorous exercise for at least 1 hour before the test.
4. If requested by a referring physician, conduct oscillometry before traditional pulmonary function tests, such as spirometry.
5. Instruct the patient to abstain from using bronchodilators before testing, unless specifically advised by a referring physician to continue such medication.

EQUIPMENT/MATERIALS PREPARATION

1. Equipment Preparation

Calibrating an oscillometry device is an important process to ensure its accuracy and reliability in measuring various parameters, typically related to oscillations or vibrations. This procedure includes assessing measurements of the device against a recognized standard or reference to recognize and correct any disparities. While we can provide you with a general overview of the calibration process, it is important to consult the specific manufacturer's guidelines and documentation for your oscillometry device, as calibration methods can vary between different devices.

Here is a basic outline of the calibration process for an oscillometry device:

Preparation: Verify that the device is functioning correctly, free from any damage, and clean. Prepare the necessary calibration standards and equipment.

Select calibration standards: Depending on the type of oscillometry device and the parameters it measures, you will need appropriate calibration standards. These standards should cover the range of measurements your device is designed for.

Perform initial check: Before calibration, perform a basic check to ensure the device is functioning properly. This could involve verifying power sources, connections, and basic functions.

Comparison to reference standard: Compare the measurements taken by your oscillometry device to those of a reference standard. The reference standard should be highly accurate and traceable to a national or international standard.

Adjustment or correction: If discrepancies are found between the device's measurements and the reference standard, adjustments might be necessary. Some devices allow for manual adjustments, while others might require professional calibration services.

Recording data: Keep detailed records of the measurements and adjustments made during the calibration process. This documentation is crucial for maintaining the device's traceability and ensuring its ongoing accuracy.

Validation: After adjustments, perform additional measurements to validate that the calibration was successful. These measurements should be consistent with the reference standard within an acceptable margin of error.

Final documentation: Once the calibration is completed and validated, generate a calibration certificate or report. This document should include information about the device, the reference standards used, the calibration process, adjustments made, and the results.

Regular calibration: Calibrating the oscillometry device is not a one-time task. Depending on usage and manufacturer recommendations, regular recalibration might be necessary. Establish a calibration schedule to ensure the device's accuracy over time.

Compliance: If your oscillometry device is used in regulated industries (such as medical or scientific applications), compliance with relevant standards and regulations might be required. Ensure that your calibration process aligns with these requirements.

Remember that the specifics of the calibration process can vary widely based on the type of oscillometry device you are using. Always refer to the manufacturer's instructions and guidelines for accurate and appropriate calibration procedures. If you are unsure about any step of the process, it is a good idea to consult with experts or professionals in the field of calibration or metrology.

2. Preparation of Materials

1. Ensure the availability of multiple 'single-patient-use-bacterial/viral' filters and nose clips.
2. Have personal protective equipment (PPE), including gloves and masks, as well as disinfectant wipes, on hand.

Minimal instructions for subjects before performing oscillometry.

- Inform the patient about the duration of a single acquisition and the anticipated number of replicates.
- Explain the sensations associated with pressure oscillations, such as a gentle "vibration" or "fluttering" in the mouth and chest during measurement.
- Consider a practice run, especially for young children.
- Encourage relaxation and "normal breathing".
- Clarify that a brief observation period precedes oscillation onset to ensure stable breathing.
- Emphasize the importance of an upright posture, with a slight "chin-up" position if seated (which should be the case for most clinical tests in adults and young children).
- Advise against swallowing during the procedure.
- Instruct and demonstrate the correct way to grip the mouthpiece with teeth and lips to prevent leaks.
- Request the patient to keep the tongue relaxed below the mouthpiece without blocking the orifice.
- If needed, instruct and demonstrate support for the cheeks and the floor of the mouth, with children receiving support from staff or parents.

Testing Procedure

1. Setting up the Oscillometry Device

1. Affix a 'single-patient-use-bacterial/viral' filter to the oscillometry device.
2. Ensure that the oscillometry device is prepared and in the testing mode.

2. Spectral Measurement

1. Remind the patient about the 30-second duration of the test and the necessity for a minimum of three measurements.
2. Direct the patient to do a nose clip and follow the provided instructions.
3. Align the oscillometry device to the patient's head level.
4. Advise the patient to moisten their lips before creating a proper, secure seal around the mouthpiece. Instruct the patient to commence normal breathing.
   Note: Check for potential air leaks around the mouthpiece and nose clip. Ensure supplementary oxygen is turned off during measurements to prevent any drift with the oscillometry device.
5. Monitor the patient's breathing pattern and start recording after observing at least three consistent tidal breaths.
   Note: (Optional): Keep the patient informed of the remaining time during each measurement, if desired.

6. Allow sufficient rest time between each measurement, adjusting as necessary based on the individual patient.
   Note: Patients using supplemental oxygen may require extended rest intervals. Administer supplemental oxygen as necessary during these breaks.
7. After completing a minimum of three measurements, assess adherence to the specified acceptability and reproducibility criteria outlined below.

3. Post-bronchodilator Response–Optional

1. Administer the bronchodilator using a spacer.
2. Record the method and quantity of doses administered.
3. Wait for 10 min post-administration of bronchodilator.
4. Repeat the above steps to assess post-bronchodilator response.

QUALITY CONTROL: CRITERIA FOR TEST ACCEPTANCE

Ensuring the accuracy of impedance measurements is crucial, and the prevention of artifacts like coughing, glottis closure, leaks, etc. is essential. To achieve this, quality control procedures must be in place to detect common artifacts such as leaks, swallows, coughs, and incorrect tongue placement. The real-time display of volume, flow, and pressure traces enables the operator to identify artifact presence, often necessitating the repetition of acquisitions until a minimum of three artifact-free measurements is obtained.[1,2]

Artifact Identification

Subjective quality control criteria involve confirming the stability of tidal volumes and rates during acquisition, as well as ensuring the absence of pauses in the volume signal accompanied by zero flow, abrupt changes, or spikes in resistance and pressure. These anomalies may indicate swallowing, breath-holds, glottic closures, or mouth leaks.[3]

Use of Coherence

Coherence can be understood as a causality index indicating the relationship between the input (flow) to the respiratory system and its "linearly" dependent output (pressure), or vice versa. Coherence values fall within the range of 0 (indicating no causality) to 1 (representing perfect causality). However, values below 0.90 or 0.95 were commonly excluded.

Quality Control/Quality Assurance

1. Conduct routine audits, scheduled either weekly or monthly based on the oscillometry testing volume in the laboratory.
2. Evaluate each operator using a standardized checklist to verify the accurate and professional execution of oscillometry tests.
3. Provide consistent feedback to operators and organize regular quality assurance meetings to address laboratory-related matters.
4. Ensure that biologic quality controls are performed weekly, involving at least two healthy non-smoking subjects, with measurements falling within ±2 SD of their mean baseline.
   Note: This is especially critical for validating testing equipment and procedures when multiple oscillometry devices are present in the laboratory.
5. Undertake quarterly self-inspections and annual factory maintenance of oscillometry devices for calibration and quality assurance checks.

Disinfection

1. Dispose of the patient's mouthpiece and nose clip in the wastebin.
2. Utilize disinfectant wipes to cleanse the oscillometry device and the patient's chair.
3. Remove gloves and sanitize hands.

   Note: Infection control policies may vary among laboratories.

Reference Values

Various published values exist for different populations, encompassing both children and adults.[4] Similar to all lung function tests, each laboratory should assess the suitability of predicted equations for a specific oscillometric device within its target population. Obtaining normative values, including bronchodilator responses, for children and adults from diverse countries requires standardized breathing protocols and signal analyses. This approach aims to derive multiethnic normative values comparable to the Global Lung Function Initiative values for spirometry.[5]

Discussion

The essential components of a high-quality oscillometry measurement fall into three domains: Patient, equipment, and operator. Key to success is ensuring the patient is in a relaxed and comfortable state, allowing measurements to be taken at resting functional residual volume. Proper patient posture is crucial, with emphasis on sitting upright, both feet on the ground, and no leg crossing. Enforcing cheek and jaw support, correct placement of the nose clip, and ensuring a sealed lip connection around the mouthpiece are vital to eliminate shunting and air leaks.[1–3] Calibration and verification of equipment must precede its use. Operators should be capable of distinguishing acceptable and unacceptable recordings, troubleshooting the root cause of undesirable readings or artifacts to guarantee reported measurements have a CoV ≤10%.[1–3] Maintenance of quality control and assurance is imperative not only for validating the oscillometry device but also for ensuring the overall quality of tests.[6–8]

Providing operators with training to identify patterns resulting from common artifacts like swallowing, leaks, and shunting enables them to promptly repeat measurements, ensuring the acquisition of high-quality tests. In cases where oscillometry is conducted at varied lung volumes, such as in the supine position, the protocol's described steps remain applicable. It is crucial to recognize that reference data, usually collected from seated subjects, may not be valid if the patient assumes a different position during the measurement.

Although oscillometry offers a quicker and simpler approach to pulmonary function testing, inaccuracies in measurements and subsequent interpretation may arise if there are deviations from the established protocol and quality control procedures. The protocol provided is tailored to the device employed in our centre, and the execution of oscillometry remains consistent across various devices. Nevertheless, variations in technical calibration and software applications may exist. Readers are encouraged to consult the manual specific to their respective instruments for guidance.

Oscillometry presents a faster and more straightforward alternative to spirometry. Additionally, individuals, including young children and adults facing language, physical, or cognitive challenges hindering the execution of forced expiratory maneuvers required in spirometry, can still undergo oscillometry, since it is conducted during natural breathing. In certain healthcare centers, oscillometry has replaced spirometry as the primary screening tool for lung diseases. Expanding training on oscillometry practices will facilitate its broader utilization as a diagnostic tool and ensure the quality control of administered tests.

Despite its speed and simplicity, oscillometry requires quality controls to guarantee precise and replicable measurements. Adhering to international guidelines enables the appropriate interpretation of research and clinical oscillometry data, allowing findings to be applicable across diverse patient populations.[9–11]

REFERENCES

1. Bates, JH, Irvin, CG, Farre, R, Hantos Z. Oscillation mechanics of the respiratory system. *Comprehensive Physiology*. 2011;1(3),1233–1272.
2. King, GG, et al. Technical standards for respiratory oscillometry. *European Respiratory Journal*. 2020;55(2), 1900753.
3. Wu, J, et al. Development of quality assurance and quality control guidelines for respiratory oscillometry in clinical studies. *Respiratory Care*. 2020;65(11),1687–1693.
4. Oostveen, E, et al. Respiratory impedance in healthy subjects: baseline values and bronchodilator response. *European Respiratory Journal*. 2013;42(6),1513–1523.
5. Brown, NJ, et al. Reference equations for respiratory system resistance and reactance in adults. *Respiratory Physiology and Neurobiology*. 2010;172(3),162–168.
6. Nowowiejska, B, et al. Transient reference values for impulse oscillometry for children aged 3-18 years. *Pediatric Pulmonology*. 2008;43(12),1193–1197.
7. Horowitz JG, Siegel SD, Primiano FP, et al. Computation of respiratory impedance from forced sinusoidal oscillations during breathing. *Comput Biomed Res* 1983; 16:499521.
8. Daróczy B, Hantos Z. Generation of optimum pseudorandom signals for respiratory impedance measurements. *Int J Biomed Comput* 1990; 25: 2131.
9. Robinson PD, Turner M, Brown NJ, et al. Procedures to improve the repeatability of forced oscillation measurements in school-aged children. *Respir Physiol Neurobiol* 2011; 177: 199206.
10. Kalchiem-Dekel O, Hines SE. Forty years of reference values for respiratory system impedance in adults: 1977 2017. *Respir Med* 2018; 136: 3747.
11. Quanjer PH, Stanojevic S, Cole TJ, et al. Multi-ethnic reference values for spirometry for the 395-year age range: the global lung function 2012 equations. *Eur Respir J* 2012; 40: 13241343.

Nomogram in Lung Oscillometry

• Thomas Vadakkan • Nishanth PS

Mechanical properties of the respiratory system (upper and intrathoracic airways, lung tissue and chest wall) during quiet tidal breathing can be measured by lung oscillometry (also known as the forced oscillation technique). An oscillating pressure signal is applied at the mouth to superimpose sound waves with normal tidal breathing. With increased clinical and research use of lung oscillometry, testing protocols will become transparent and thereby allowing standardization, comparison, and replication of clinical and research studies and methodologies.

An updated list of predicted impedance values in adults and children for lung oscillometry was provided by ERS technical standards for respiratory oscillometry published in 2020.[1]

Normal Graph

Figure 4.1 showing in relationship between resistance or reactance with oscillation frequency.

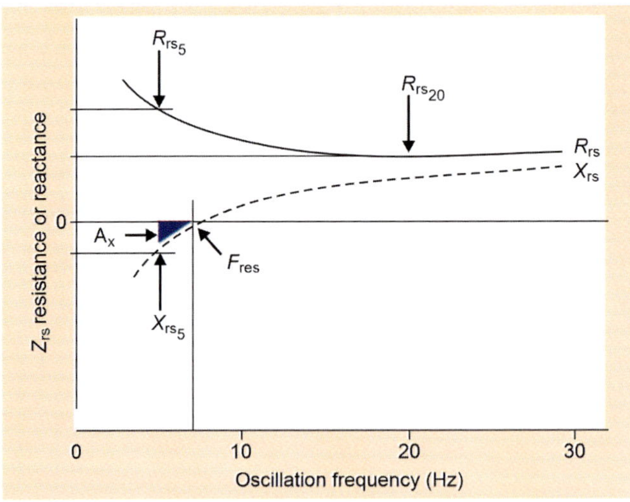

Fig. 4.1: Relationship between resistance or reactance with oscillation frequency

NORMAL HEALTHY SUBJECTS

The oscillogram and parameters of lung oscillometry from a healthy adult subject are typically characterized by an almost flat resistance curve. While age and height dependent, the values for R_5 should be ≤2.0 to 3.0 cmH$_2$O.s/L. There is very minimal frequency dependence of resistance; hence, the R_{5-20} is close to 0, which indicates the absence of small airway disease in healthy normal adults. The X_5 of the reactance curve is typically ≥2.0 and the F_{res} between 8 and 12 Hz. A$_x$ is <10 cmH$_2$O/L in normal healthy adults.

Following parameters are important in interpreting lung oscillometry

1. The R_5 is the resistance of the total respiratory system from mouth to body surface. Normal value of R_5 should be ≤2.0 to 3.0 cmH$_2$O.s/L. It should be lower than 150% of R_5 pred (FOT-4)
2. R_{20} is the resistance of the proximal airway. Normal value of R_{20} should be lower than 150% of R_{20} pred (FOT-3).
3. (R_{5-20}) is a sensitive measure of small airway dysfunction (SAD) and helps to diagnose SAD asthma confidently in our day-to-day practice. In Morbid obesity, lung oscillometry may show SAD pattern due to distal airway resistance.[2-7]
4. The reactance at 5 Hz (X_5) measures the elastic, or stiffness properties of the respiratory system. In peripheral airway obstruction and restrictive lung disease X_5 is more negative.[8-10]
5. At a particular frequency, the capacitative and inertive pressure components are equal and are opposite in phase with each other, therefore, the total reactance at this frequency is zero. This frequency is called the resonant frequency (F_{res}). Normal values of F_{res} in adults range from 7 to 12 Hz.[11] F_{res} and resistance are inversely proportional to age: They tend to be higher in younger children and lower in older children and adults. F_{res} may be elevated in both restrictive and obstructive disorders.
6. Reactance area (AX) provides information about the smaller airways (from the 8th to 23rd generation of the airways). It represents total reactance at all frequencies between 5 Hz and the resonant frequency. The normal AX is <10 cmH$_2$O/L.[12]

Shape of the Oscillogram in Normal Individuals (Fig. 4.2)

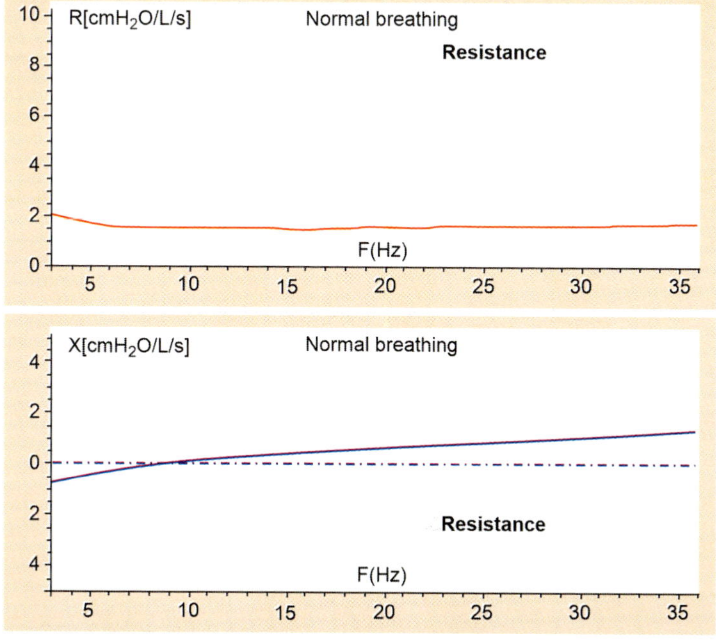

Fig. 4.2: Shape of the oscillogram in normal individuals during tidal breathing

REFERENCES

1. Dubois A, Brody A, Lewis D, et al. Oscillation mechanics of lungs and chest in man. J Appl Physiol 1956;8:587–94.
2. Foy BH, Soares M, Bordas R, et al. Lung computational models and the role of the small airways in asthma. Am J Respir Crit Care Med. 2019. doi:10.1164/rccm.201812-2322OC.
3. Kaczka DW, Lutchen KR, Hantos Z. Emergent behavior of regional heterogeneity in the lung and its effects on respiratory impedance. J Appl Physiol. 2011;110:1473–81. doi:10.1152/japplphysiol.01287.2010
4. Desager KN, Cauberghs M, Naudts J, et al. Influence of upper airway shunt on total respiratory impedance in infants. J Appl Physiol.1999;87:902–09. doi:10.1152/jappl.1999.87.3.902.72.
5. Bates JH, Allen GB. The estimation of lung mechanics parameters in the presence of pathology: a theoretical analysis. Ann Biomed Eng. 2006;34:384–92. doi:10.1007/s10439-005-9056-6.73.
6. Bhatawadekar SA, Leary D, Maksym GN. Modelling resistance and reactance with heterogeneous airway narrowing in mild to severe asthma. Can J Physiol Pharmacol. 2015;93:207–14. doi:10.1139/cjpp-2014-0436.74.
7. Cauberghs M, Van De Woestijne KP. Effect of upper airway shunt and series properties on respiratory impedance measurements. J Appl Physiol. 1989;66:2274–79. doi:10.1152/jappl.1989.66.5.2274.75.
8. Albuquerque CG, de Andrade FMD, de Rocha MA, de A, et al. Determining respiratory system resistance and reactance by impulse oscillometry in obese individuals. J Bras Pneumol. 2015;41:422–26. doi:10.1590/S1806-37132015000004517.
9. Naglaa BA, Kamal E. Role of IOS in evaluation of patients with interstitial lung diseases. Egypt J Chest Dis Tuberc. 2016;65:791–95. doi:10.1016/j.ejcdt.2016.05.002.
10. Dandurand R, Dandurand M, Estepar R, et al. Oscillometry in community practice ild is characterized by abnormal reactance but normal resistance. Quart J Med. 2016;109:S50. doi:10.1093/qjmed/hcw127.019.32.
11. Hogg JC, Williams J, Richardson JB, Macklem PT, Thurlbeck WM. Age as a factor in the distribution of lower-airway conductance and in the pathologic anatomy of obstructive lung disease. N Engl J Med 1970;282:1283–7.
12. Eddy RL, Westcott A, Maksym GN, et al. Oscillometry and pulmonary magnetic resonance imaging in asthma and COPD. Physiol Rep. 2019;7:e13955. doi:10.14814/phy2.13955.

Spirometry Versus Oscillometry

• *Manju Rajaram*

Pulmonary function testing (PFT) is important for diagnosing and monitoring lung diseases which include obstructive and restrictive lung disease. Spirometry is more commonly used in regular practice and it is one of the standard diagnostic tests for lung disease. For different ethnicities, anthropometry-matched reference values were available. Even though with standardization, only 21% of physicians use this procedure, but it is very difficult to do in most of the individuals like children, elderly and, neuromuscular disease patients because of the forceful maneuvers. And it requires patient cooperation. Oscillometry diagnostic test is a non-invasive and well-researched technique. It allows passive measurement of lung mechanics by tidal breathing. So, it does not require forceful inspiratory and expiratory maneuvers.[1]

Even though oscillometry is not given in asthma and COPD management guidelines, it will detect small airway changes earlier compared to spirometry.[2] Still whether oscillometry will replace spirometry in airway disease is questionable. This chapter aims to compare spirometry and oscillometry, outlining indications, contraindications, advantages, and limitations. Understanding the distinct features of these tests is essential for optimal clinical decision-making and patient care.

SPIROMETRY

Principle

Spirometry is a widely recognized and standard lung function test utilized to measure the lung function, which measures the maximum volume of air that a person can inhale and exhale with full effort. The primary signal recorded during spirometry is either the volume of air or the flow of air, both of which are tracked over time. This test provides essential information about lung health and is commonly used to diagnose and monitor respiratory conditions.[3]

Indications

Spirometry is indicated in the following situations.

Diagnosis

1. Evaluation of signs and symptom
2. Measuring the effect of disease
3. Screening the people who have the risk of pulmonary disease

4. Preoperative evaluation
5. Prognosis assessment

Monitoring

1. To assess the response of therapeutic intervention
2. Monitoring the progression of disease
3. To assess the adverse effects of injurious agents exposure
4. Watching for adverse reactions of drug.

Disability/Impairment Evaluations

1. Assessing the effect of rehabilitation program
2. Assessing the risks as part of an insurance evaluation
3. Assessing individuals for legal reasons.

Others

1. Clinical trials
2. Epidemiological surveys
3. Reference equations derivation
4. Pre-employment and lung health monitoring for at-risk occupations
5. Assessing health status before beginning at-risk physical activities.

Relative Contraindications for Spirometry[4,5]

Due to increases in myocardial demand or changes in blood pressure
1. Acute myocardial infarction within 1 week
2. Systemic hypotension or severe hypertension
3. Significant atrial/ventricular arrhythmia
4. Non-compensated heart failure
5. Uncontrolled pulmonary hypertension
6. Acute cor pulmonale
7. Clinically unstable pulmonary embolism
8. History of syncope related to forced expiration/cough

Due to increases in intracranial/intraocular pressure[6]
1. Cerebral aneurysm
2. Brain surgery within 4 weeks
3. Recent concussion with continuing symptoms
4. Eye surgery within 1 week

Due to increases in sinus and middle ear pressures
1. Sinus surgery or middle ear surgery or infection within 1 week.

Due to increases in intrathoracic and intra-abdominal pressure[7]
1. Presence of pneumothorax
2. Thoracic surgery within 4 weeks
3. Abdominal surgery within 4 weeks
4. Late-term pregnancy

Infection control issues

1. Active respiratory or systemic infection, which includes tuberculosis
2. Conditions which causing transmission of infections, like hemoptysis.

Variables Use in Spirometry[3]

Variable	Unit
FVC	Litre
FEV_1	Litre
FEV_1/FVC	Decimal fraction
PEF	Litre/second
FET	Second
FIVC	Litre
Children <6 years	
FEV 0.75	Litre
FEV 0.75/FVC	Decimal fraction

Spirometry Analysis[8]

It begins with evaluating the ratio of forced expiratory volume in 1 second (FEV_1) to vital capacity (VC). Traditionally, the FEV_1 to forced vital capacity (FVC) ratio (FEV_1/FVC%) was used to differentiate between obstructive disorders, normal lung function, or restrictive diseases. However, the ATS/ERS recommends to use the FVC, slow vital capacity (SVC), or forced inspiratory vital capacity (FIVC) as the denominator, whichever yields the greatest value. If the FEV_1/VC ratio is below the lower limit of normal (LLN) (i.e. below the fifth percentile), and the vital capacity ≥LLN, an obstructive pattern is identified. On the other hand, if the total lung capacity (TLC) is ≤ LLN, a mixed pattern is suggested. To distinguish between asthma and emphysema, the diffusing capacity of the lung for carbon monoxide (DLCO) is examined, being normal in asthma or chronic bronchitis and reduced in emphysema (Fig. 5.1).

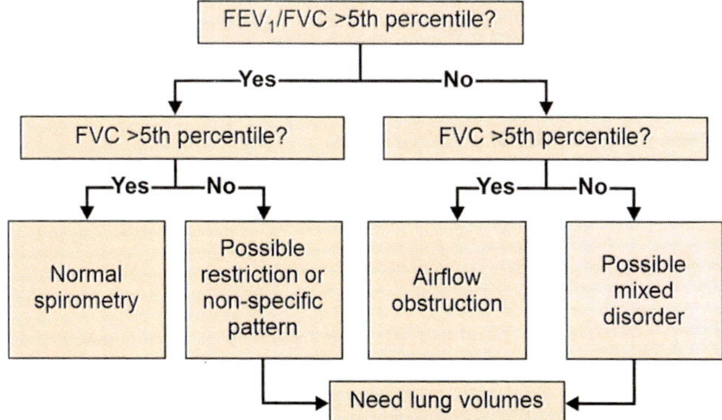

Fig. 5.1: Approach to interpretation of spirometry

Advantages[9]

- Spirometry is a well-established and standardised test used in clinical practice and research.
- It provides essential parameters that aid in the diagnosis and classification of various lung disorders.
- The test is relatively simple, non-invasive, and easily reproducible.
- It helps in risk stratification and guiding therapeutic decisions in respiratory diseases.

Limitations[10]

- Spirometry relies on cooperation of patient and patient effort, which may be challenging in certain patient populations, such as young children, elderly individuals, or those with cognitive impairments.
- It provides limited information on small airways function, as it primarily assesses larger airway flows.
- Spirometry may not be sensitive enough to find out the early or subtle changes in pulmonary function.

OSCILLOMETRY

Oscillometry, also known as forced oscillation technique (FOT), is a non-invasive test and independent of effort. It provides information regarding the mechanical properties of the lung parenchyma, larger and the smaller airways.[11]

Based on the oscillation signal types, oscillometry classified into the following types:[12]

1. **Monofrequency oscillometry:** This type uses a single sinusoidal pressure waveform to assess lung function. It is particularly used for patients monitoring with sleep apnea or those receiving mechanical ventilatory support, such as continuous positive airway pressure (CPAP).
2. **Pseudorandom noise (PRN) oscillometry:** PRN oscillometry involves applying impulses of several frequencies simultaneously. This type of oscillometry is most commonly used for assessing the obstructive lung diseases like asthma and COPD, as well as restrictive lung diseases such as interstitial lung disease, and thoracic wall deformities.
3. **Impulse oscillometry (IOS):** In this type of oscillometry, recurrent impulses in the form of a square form at frequency of 5 Hz. IOS is a specific method of oscillometry that is used to assess lung function and respiratory mechanics in clinical practice and research settings (Fig. 5.2A and B).

Various Terminologies of Oscillatory Mechanic[13]

Respiratory impedance analysis parameters in forced oscillation technique (FOT) (Fig. 5.3A and B).

1. **Impedance (Z):** It represents the total sum of inertial, resistive, and elastic forces encountered by a pressure impulse during its passage through the pulmonary system. It is calculated by a combination of resistance (R) and reactance (X), where R is a real force and X is an imaginary component associated with energy storage and dissipation.

$$Z(\omega) = R(\omega) + jX(\omega)$$

(j is the unit imaginary number represented as $\sqrt{-1}$)

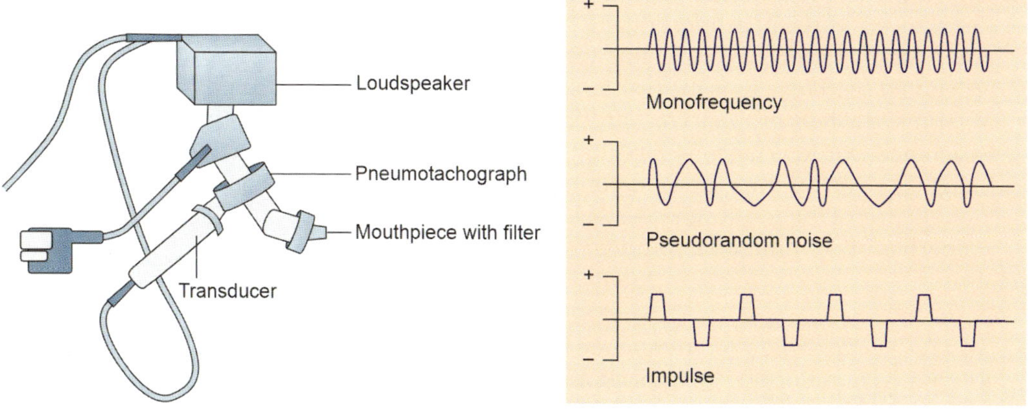

Fig. 5.2A and B: Impulse oscillometry

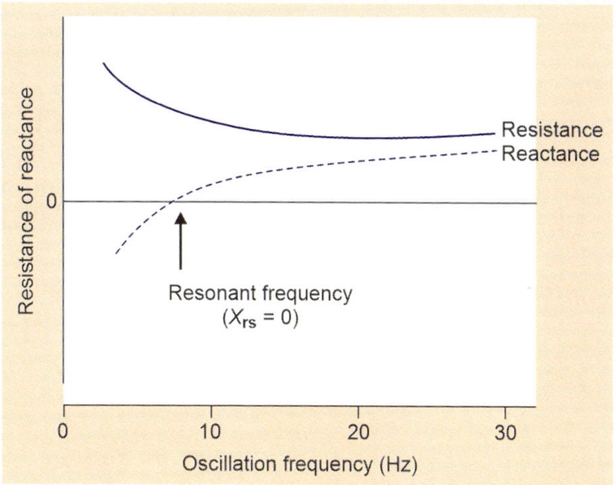

Fig. 5.3A

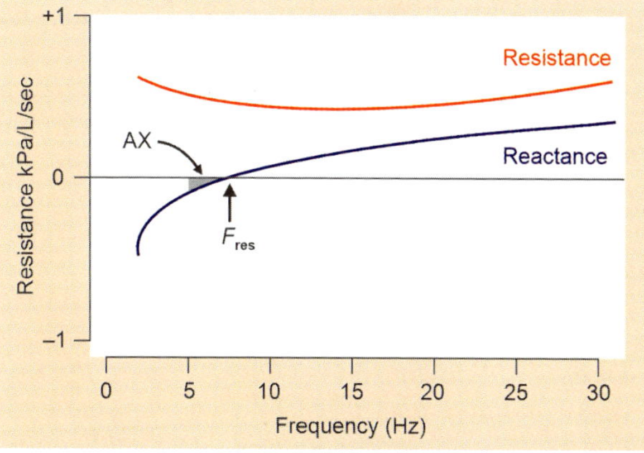

Fig. 5.3B

2. **Resistance (R):** Resistance is a measure of opposition to airflow in the respiratory system. Resistance is directly proportional to the length and inversely proportional to the fourth power of the radius of conducting tubes. Resistance expressed at a specific frequency (f) is denoted as Rf (e.g. R_5 is the resistance measured at 5 Hz). Rf encompasses the resistance of larynx, trachea, oropharynx, large and small airways, lungs, and chest wall.

3. **Reactance (X):** Reactance is rebound resistance created by distensible airways. It is an imaginary part of impedance determined by the balance between capacitance (C) and inertance (I) of the respiratory system. Capacitance is inversely correlated with the elastic properties of the pulmonary system.

$$X(\omega) = \omega.I - E/\omega$$
$$X(\omega) = \omega.I - 1/\omega.C$$

(where ω is the oscillation frequency function)

4. **Resonant frequency (F_{res}):** Capacitative and inertial forces are equal at specific frequency which results in zero reactance. Below F_{res}, elastic forces is predominant, whereas above F_{res}, inertance of airway plays a main role. Resonant frequency is more in childhood and decreases with age.

5. **Reactance area (A_x):** It is the triangular area between F_{res} and reactance at 5 Hz. A_x gives information about distal airways and parenchyma. It is a sensitive parameter for detecting small airway obstruction and documenting bronchodilator reversibility.

6. **Coherence:** Coherence is a quality control variable that reflects the reliability of the oscillometry maneuver. It is based on the difference between the input (flow) and output (reflected pressure) in the pulmonary system. Higher coherence values indicate satisfactory maneuver quality. However, different manufacturers may use different approaches for calculations, leading to differing coherence values.

7. **Coefficient of variation (CoV%):** CoV% is another quality control parameter used to assess the reliability of the measurements. A CoV% ≤10% in adults and ≤15% in children for two sets of R_5 is considered acceptable.

Clinical Implications[14]

1. **Clinical lung function laboratories:** Oscillometry is frequently utilized in clinical lung function laboratories to complement traditional pulmonary function tests such as spirometry, different lung volumes, and diffusing capacity of lung parenchyma. It provides additional insights into respiratory impedance, resistance, reactance, and resonant frequency, particularly in individuals who may have difficulty in doing spirometry in view of poor cooperation or frailty.

2. **Field testing:** Oscillometry can be used in field testing to assess respiratory function in a non-clinical setting, making it a practical tool for large population studies and occupational health screening. Its less testing times and ease of administration make it advantageous for such studies.

3. **Home monitoring:** Self-operated daily oscillometry in home has been shown to be practical in patients with chronic obstructive pulmonary disease (COPD) and asthma. This approach allows for the collection of daily data, enabling calculation of day-to-day variability and potential clinical use for diagnosis, therapy response monitoring, and clinical phenotyping.

4. **Pediatric lung diseases:** Oscillometry finds widespread clinical application in pediatric lung diseases. It is particularly useful in children who have difficulty performing spirometry at a young age. Oscillometry can provide valuable information about airway resistance and reactance in pediatric patients with various respiratory conditions.

5. **Intensive care unit (ICU):** Oscillometry can be utilized to optimise mechanical ventilation in the ICU or operating room. It offers potential benefits in monitoring patients on mechanical ventilation and optimising ventilation strategies.

Advantages[15]

- Oscillometry is less effort-dependent than spirometry, making it suitable for young children, older patients, and patient with physical limitations.
- Oscillometry provides detailed information on the small airways' function, which is not captured adequately by spirometry.
- The test is well-tolerated and can be performed quickly.
- This test is independent of height, age and sex.

Limitations[16]

- Oscillometry is less standardized and less commonly used in clinical practice than spirometry.
- The interpretation of oscillometry parameters can be complex and requires expertise.
- It may not provide all the parameters required for definitive diagnosis or disease classification.

Clinical Solution that Oscillometry Address[17]

Issue with Spirometry

- Spirometry requires forceful maneuvers, requires patient co-operation.
- Children with less than 5 years, older people and those with physically challenged and patient with cognitive limitations cannot perform spirometry.
- Pre- and post-bronchodilator testing with forced flow-volume loops maneuvers and body plethysmography are difficult to perform by many patients especially in acute exacerbation COPD patients. Forceful inhalation will alter the bronchial spasm in COPD and asthma in adults and childhood.
- Even though with varied application of airways clearance techniques (ACTs) in pulmonary rehabilitation, objective outcome measurement for these patients could not be measure using spirometry.

Oscillometry Solutions

- Easy to perform test, 10 breaths tidal breathing testing mode for obstruction identification and localization, automatic rejection of non-physiological breath, for quality control.
- Pre- and post-bronchodilator testings are easy to evaluate results and improvement. Oscillometry has considerable advantage that it measures airway properties during quiet breathing, make it repeatable and reliable on all subjects. Inspiratory resistance and reactance at 5 Hz. It allows objective measurement and quantification of ACT.

SPIROMETRY VERSUS OSCILLOMETRY (Table 5.1)

- Spirometry needs a well-trained technician. While performing spirometry, the technician has to teach the procedure properly to the subject and has to continuously encourage the subject to get valid, reliable and reproducible results. It cannot be done in children or elderly. We have valid reference equations based on age, height, sex and race. Reference

TABLE 5.1: Spirometry and oscillometry (FOT/IOS)[1]

	Spirometry	*Oscillometry*
Principle	Flow sensor/volume displacement helps in measuring flow rates and volumes of lung	Forced oscillations of single frequency (FOT) or impulses of multiple frequency sound waves (IOS) are pushed into the lungs as pressure waves to measure respiratory resistance and reactance
Variables	FEV_1 and FVC Flows: PEFR, $FEF_{25-75\%}$	Z_{rs}, R_{rs}, X_{rs}, F_{res}, A_x
Patient cooperation required	+++	+
Types of breathing maneuver	Forced exhalation	Tidal breathing
Variability	3–5%	5–15%
Sensitivity to airway location		
Central	+	+++
Peripheral	++	+++
Cut off for bronchodilator response	10–20% for FEV_1	40% for R_5 or X_5
Cut off for bronchoconstrictor response	20% for FEV_1	50% for R_5
Insight into lung mechanics	+	+++
Standardized methodology	+++	++
Availability of robust reference values	+++	+

FEV_1: Forced expiratory volume in 1s; FVC: Forced vital capacity; PEFR: Peak expiratory flow rate; $FEF_{25-75\%}$ of FVC; Z_{rs}: Respiratory impedance, R_{rs}: respiratory resistance, X_{rs}: respiratory reactance, F_{res}: resonant frequency, A_x: Reactance area; R_5: Respiratory resistance at 5 Hz; X_5; Respiratory reactance at 5 Hz

equations are available for almost all races. This procedure is standardized. Standard algorithms and diagnostic criteria are available for diagnosis and for bronchial challenge and reversibility testing. The severity of the condition can be assessed. However, the normal range of $FEF_{25-75\%}$ is very large which makes diagnosis of small airway disease/dysfunction difficult. Finally, the equipment is cheap and portable.

- Impulse oscillometry, on the other hand, does not need adequate training of the technician or the subject. It can be done even in an infant. The results are easily reproducible. However, we do not have reference equations which can be applied globally. With respect to India, adequate studies are not available to form reference equations. Early diagnosis of obstructive airway disease or restrictive lung disease can be done with IOS enabling early intervention. The diagnosis of small airway disease/dysfunction can be made with certainty with IOS. However, the severity cannot be assessed. As compared to spirometry, IOS is preferable for reversibility testing and provocation testing. The required dose of provocating agent is very less in IOS, making it a safer procedure. Studies done in ICU settings are also showing promising results regarding the applicability of IOS for adjusting the ventilatory settings. Finally, the equipment is costly as compared to spirometer.

CONCLUSION

Both spirometry and oscillometry are valuable tools in assessing lung function. Spirometry is a well-established and widely used test, providing essential parameters for diagnosing and managing various lung diseases. On the other hand, oscillometry is a technique which is slowly gaining fame and acceptance all over the world. It offers unique insights into small airway function and is particularly useful in patients who cannot perform spirometry reliably. The choice between these tests depends on the clinical context, the patient's ability to cooperate, and the specific lung function parameters needed for evaluation. In many cases, a combination of both spirometry and oscillometry can provide a more comprehensive assessment of lung function, enabling better patient care and management of respiratory conditions. Studies need to be done all over the world to get valid predicted values for each of the parameters of oscillometry.

REFERENCES

1. Brashier B, Salvi S. Measuring lung function using sound waves: role of the forced oscillation technique and impulse oscillometry system. Breathe [Internet]. 2015;11:57–65.
2. Li LY, Yan TS, Yang J, Li YQ, Fu LX, Lan L, et al. Impulse oscillometry for detection of small airway dysfunction in subjects with chronic respiratory symptoms and preserved pulmonary function. Respir Res. 2021;22:68.
3. Graham BL, Steenbruggen I, Miller MR, Barjaktarevic IZ, Cooper BG, Hall GL, et al. Standardization of Spirometry 2019 Update. An Official American Thoracic Society and European Respiratory Society Technical Statement. Am J Respir Crit Care Med. 2019;200:e70–88.
4. Cooper BG. An update on contraindications for lung function testing. Thorax. 2011;66:714–23.
5. Coates AL, Graham BL, McFadden RG, McParland C, Moosa D, Provencher S, et al. Canadian Thoracic Society. Spirometry in primary care. Can Respir J 2013;20:13–21-Google Search.
6. Vieira GM, Oliveira HB, de Andrade DT, Bottaro M, Ritch R. Intraocular pressure variation during weight lifting. Arch Ophthalmol. 2006;124:1251–4.
7. Effect of spirometry on intra-thoracic pressures | BMC Research Notes | Full Text [Internet]. [cited 2023 Aug 18]. Available from: https://bmcresnotes.biomedcentral.com/articles/10.1186/s13104-018-3217-9
8. ERS/ATS technical standard on interpretive strategies for routine lung function tests | European Respiratory Society.
9. Spirometry [Internet]. nhs.uk. 2017. Available from: https://www.nhs.uk/conditions/spirometry/
10. Kolsum U, Borrill Z, Roy K, Starkey C, Vestbo J, Houghton C, et al. Impulse oscillometry in COPD: identification of measurements related to airway obstruction, airway conductance and lung volumes. Respir Med. 2009;103:136–43.
11. Saadeh C, Cross B, Saadeh C, Gaylor M. Retrospective Observations on the Ability to Diagnose and Manage Patients with Asthma through the Use of Impulse Oscillometry: Comparison with Spirometry and Overview of the Literature. Pulm Med. 2014;2014:376–890.
12. Clinical Application of the Forced Oscillation Technique – PubMed [Internet]. Available from: https://pubmed.ncbi.nlm.nih.gov/26984069/
13. Kaczka DW, Dellacá RL. Oscillation mechanics of the respiratory system: applications to lung disease. Crit Rev Biomed Eng. 2011;39:337–59.
14. King GG, Bates J, Berger KI, Calverley P, Melo PL de, Dellacà RL, et al. Technical standards for respiratory oscillometry. *European Respiratory Journal.* 2020;55.
15. Lauhkonen E, Kaltsakas G, Sivagnanasithiyar S, Iles R. Comparison of forced oscillation technique and spirometry in paediatric asthma. ERJ Open Research. 2021;7.
16. Clinical significance and applications of oscillometry | European Respiratory Society.
17. Desiraju K, Agrawal A. Impulse oscillometry: The state-of-the-art for lung function testing. Lung India. 2016;33:410–6.

Interpretation of Oscillometry

• Nishanth PS

By the technique of lung oscillometry, lung mechanics can be passively measured.[1] In lung oscillometry sound waves are superimposed on normal tidal breathing. By the technique of superimposition there will be disturbances in flow and pressure across the airways. Lung oscillometry measures respiratory resistance, reactance and impedance.[2] About the total respiratory resistance, 46% is offered by the chest wall, 20% by the nose, 20% by large- and medium-sized airways and about 7% by the small airways (from the 8th to 23rd generation of airways).

The technique of lung oscillometry is based on the Ohm's law which states that the relationship between pressure and flow tells us about airway resistance (Resistance = Pressure/Flow). Lung oscillometry is an effort independent method which involves the application of sound waves that help in calculation of resistance and reactance by measuring changes in pressure and flow across the airways.[3]

The main technical advantage of FOT/IOS is that it is effort independent, requires minimal patient cooperation and only simple tidal breathing maneuvers by the patient. Even children, elderly, patients on ventilators and also during sleep can perform FOT/IOS.[4]

FOT/IOS can be easily done in subjects who are unable to perform routine spirometry. IOS is more sensitive than spirometry for peripheral/small airway disease and can help in the efficient diagnosis of cough variant bronchial asthma and also SAD-asthma (small airway dysfunction-asthma)[5] which can help in clinical management in this subset of patients as they require nebulization with ultrafine particles.

FOT/IOS can be used especially in asthma where it can help in measuring bronchodilator response.[6] Lung oscillometry can help in the diagnosis of asthma particularly the small airway and cough variant phenotype at an earlier stage and also help in predicting poor symptom control in these subset of patients.[7]

When multiple frequencies are used, the characteristics of the different regions of the tracheobronchial tree including the central and peripheral airways can be analysed.[8] Sound waves with higher frequencies (20 Hz) provide information about the resistance (R_{20}) of the large airways, as they travel shorter distances. Sound waves with lower frequencies (5 Hz) provide information about entire tracheobronchial tree, as they travel larger distances. Therefore, the resistance at 5 Hz (R_5) represents the total airway resistance. The difference between R_5 and R_{20} (R_{5-20}) gives the resistance of the smaller airways[9] (Fig. 6.1). Frequencies higher than 20 Hz are not used as they cause discomfort and lower frequencies are not used as they get altered by breath dynamics.

The values provided by lung oscillometry include respiratory impedance (Z_{rs}), which includes respiratory resistance (R_{rs}) and respiratory reactance (X_{rs})

$$Z_{rs} = R_{rs} + X_{rs}$$

PARAMETERS THAT LUNG OSCILLOMETRY MEASURES

1. Respiratory resistance (R_{rs})
2. Respiratory reactance (X_{rs}): $I + C$ (Inertance + Capacitance)
3. Resonant frequency (F_{res})
4. Area of reactance (A_x)

1. Respiratory Resistance (R_{rs})

Respiratory resistance is frequency independent and tells us about the forward pressure or resistance offered by the airways. Respiratory resistance, 46% is offered by the chest wall, 20% by the nose, 20% by large and medium sized airways and about 7% by the small airways (from

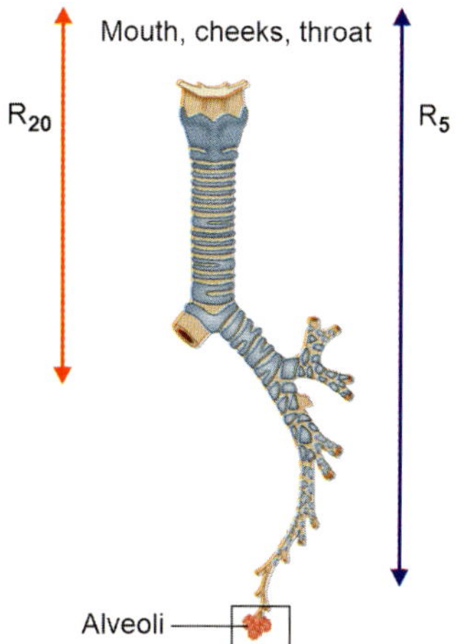

Fig. 6.1: Schematic representation of sound waves of different frequencies and their distance travelled

the 8th to 23rd generation of airways). The use of multiple oscillatory frequencies allows characterization of pure large airways obstruction from pure small airways obstruction from combined large and small airway obstruction.[11]

Sound waves of lower frequencies (5 Hz) traverse the entire airway (proximal airway + small airway) and those at higher frequencies (20 Hz) are damped out in the first 7 generations of airway, i.e. proximal airways.[12] Therefore, R_5-resistance at 5 Hz represents the total airway resistance, and R_{20} represents the pure resistance of the large/central airways. Difference between R_{5-20} provides pure small airways resistance. Resistance is independent of oscillation frequency (i.e. resistance is almost same at frequencies between 5 and 20 Hz) in healthy adults.[13]

During airways disease/obstruction either in large or small airways, R_5 is increased.[14] Airway in pure large airways obstruction, resistance increases uniformly independent of the oscillation frequencies, whereas in pure small airways obstruction increases resistance at lower frequencies (Fig. 6.2).

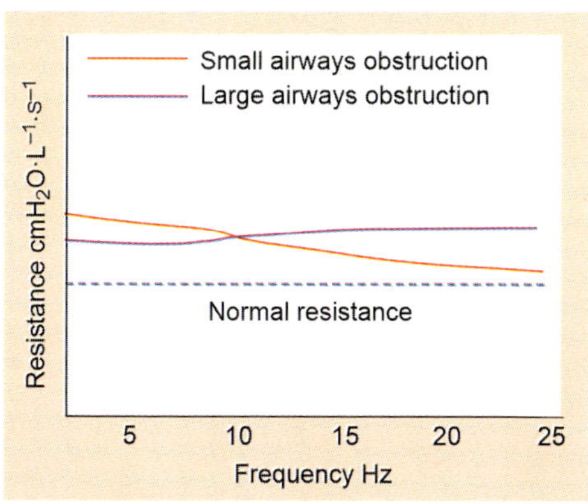

Fig. 6.2: Graphical representation of resistance vs frequency in cases of small and large airways obstruction

The characteristic feature of small airways disease is that resistance is dependent on the frequency of waves delivered.[15] In younger age group, the airway resistance is usually frequency dependent.[16] The unit of measurement of airway resistance is $cmH_2O{\cdot}L^{-1}{\cdot}s^{-1}$ or $kPa{\cdot}L^{-1}{\cdot}s^{-1}$.[17] To convert $kPa{\cdot}L^{-1}{\cdot}s^{-1}$ to $cmH_2O{\cdot}L^{-1}{\cdot}s^{-1}$ we have to multiply by 10.

2. Respiratory Reactance (X_{rs}): Inertance + Capacitance

Respiratory reactance (X_{rs}) is related to the volume changes caused by the moving column of air.

Inertive properties are related to acceleration of gas flow along lung or chest wall as they move through the air column.

Capacitance (C) is related to elasticity and compliance of the airways and is primarily located in the periphery of the lung.[18] At a particular frequency, known as the resonant frequency, capacitance (C) and inertance (I) are exactly equal and are in opposite phase with each other, so the reactance (X_{rs}) will be zero at that point. Reactance (X_{rs}) is actually the rebound resistance and gives information about the smaller airways. In FOT/IOS, by convention capacitance is negative and inertance is positive. X_5 (reactance at 5 Hz) gives information about the smaller airways and also about the tissue elastance/compliance. Resonant frequency (F_{res}) is the frequency at which the capacitance and inertance are equal, but in opposite phase with each other therefore the total reactance is zero.[19] Reactance values are measured in $cmH_2O{\cdot}L^{-1}{\cdot}s^{-1}$ or $kPa{\cdot}L^{-1}{\cdot}s^{-1}$.[20] To convert $kPa{\cdot}L^{-1}{\cdot}s^{-1}$ to $cmH_2O{\cdot}L^{-1}{\cdot}s^{-1}$ we have to multiply by 10 (Fig. 6.3).

At the lower frequency (5 Hz), in respiratory reactance, tissue elastance would predominate. Elastance, the reciprocal of compliance, is the pressure required to inflate the lungs. X_5 gives information about elastic recoil of the smaller airways, i.e. from the 8th to 23rd generation.[21,22] Conditions such as lung fibrosis and hyperinflation that reduce the compliance of the lungs will have higher X_5 values as the capacitance is more negative.[23]

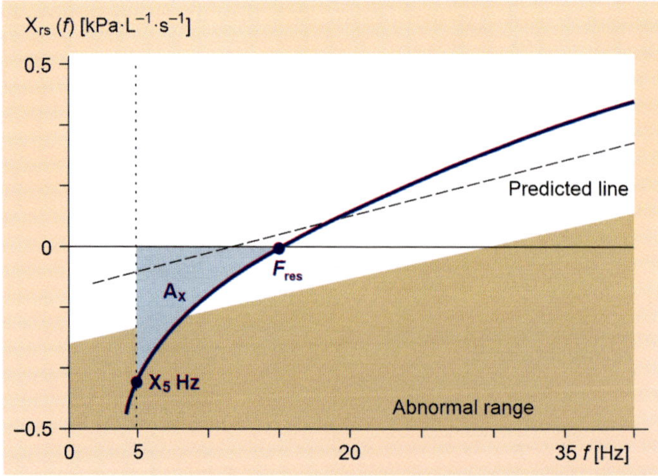

Fig. 6.3: Graphical representation showing changes in reactance (X_5) with increasing frequency. F_{res}: Resonant frequency, X_5: Reactance at 5 Hz, A_x: Area of reactance

3. Resonant Frequency (F_{res})

At a particular frequency, the capacitative and inertive pressure components are equal and are opposite in phase with each other, therefore the total reactance at this frequency is zero. This frequency is called the resonant frequency (F_{res}).

Below the resonant frequency, capacitance will predominate (negative by convention) and above the resonant frequency, inertance will predominate (positive by convention).

Normal F_{res}: 7–12 Hz. Resonant frequency increases in both obstructive and restrictive diseases. Children have higher F_{res}, decreases with age.

4. Reactance Area (A_x)/"Goldman Triangle"

Reactance area (A_x) provides information about the smaller airways (from the 8th to 23rd generation of the airways).

It represents total reactance at all frequencies between 5 Hz and the resonant frequency.

A_x is also called the "Goldman Triangle" (named after Michael Goldman who described it for the first time). It is measured in $cmH_2O \cdot L^{-1}$ or $kPa \cdot L^{-1}$.

A_x is a useful parameter that tells about the degree of small airway obstruction and also about the respiratory compliance. It is closely related with R_{5-20}. The normal A_x is generally <0.33 $kPa \cdot L^{-1}$.

INTERPRETATION IN A NUTSHELL

1. **Resistance (R):** R_5, R_{20}, and R_{5-20} represents the combined small and large airways resistance, large airway resistance, and small airway resistance respectively.

   In younger children due to significant contribution of airway resistance by smaller airways, R_{5-20} is higher in this subset of population.[24]
2. **Reactance (X):** Measured at 5 Hz and becomes more negative in both pure small airway obstruction and in restrictive lung diseases. It is not affected by pure large airway obstruction.
3. **Resonant frequency (F_{res}):** F_{res} increases (shifts to right) in both restrictive and in pure small airway obstructive airway diseases.[20] F_{res} is normal in pure large airway obstruction.
4. **Area of reactance (A_x):** A_x increases in both pure small airway obstruction and also in restrictive lung diseases.[8] It remains normal in pure large airway obstruction.

CASE SCENARIOS (Figs 6.4 to 6.6 and Table 6.1)

a. *Pure small airway obstruction:* R_5 increases, R_{5-20} increases (with normal R_{20}), X_5 becomes more negative, A_x increases.

   (*Note:* Frequency dependent airway resistance ($R \alpha 1/f$).[24]
b. *Pure large airway obstruction:* R_5 increases, R_{20} increases (with normal R_{5-20}), X_5 remains normal, A_x remains normal (frequency independent).
c. *Combined small and large airway obstruction:* R_5, R_{20}, R_{5-20}, A_x, F_{res} will be increased, X_5 will be more negative.
d. *Restrictive lung diseases:* R_5, R_{20}, R_{5-20} will be normal, X_5 will be more negative and A_x, F_{res} will be increased (Fig. 6.6).

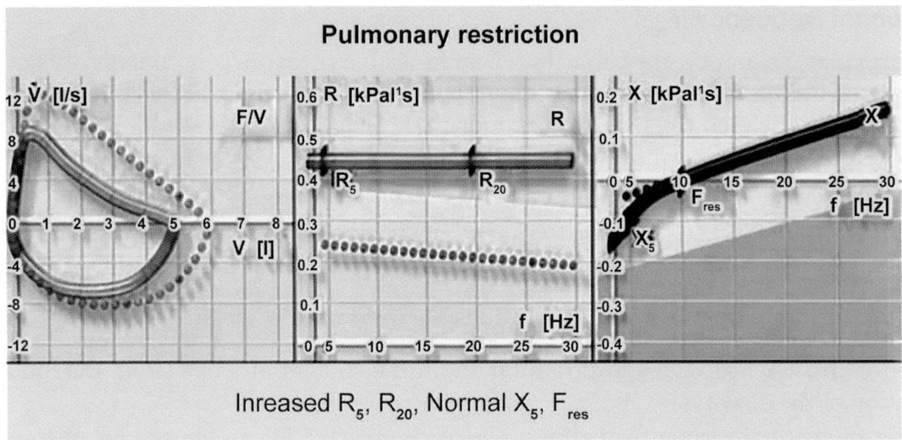

Fig. 6.4: Impulse oscillometry in proximal/central airway obstruction

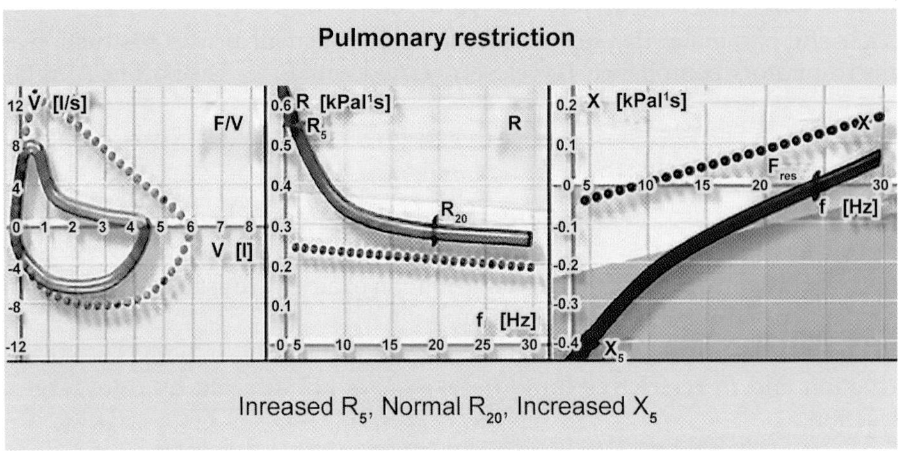

Fig. 6.5: Impulse oscillometry in peripheral airway obstruction

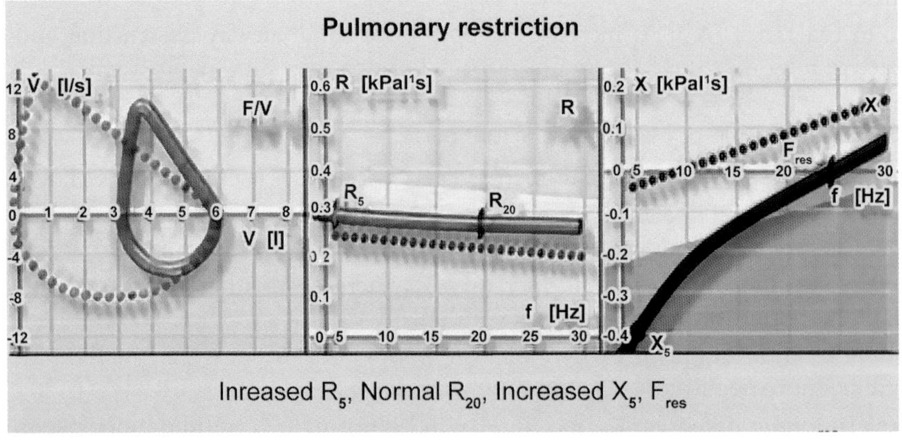

Fig. 6.6: Impulse oscillometry in restrictive airway diseases

TABLE 6.1: Interpretation of lung oscillometry parameters

Conditions	R_5	R_{20}	R_{5-20}	X_5	A_x	F_{res}
Pure small airway obstruction	↑↑↑	N	↑↑	More negative	↑↑	↑↑
Pure large airway obstruction	↑↑	↑↑	N	N	N	N
Combined small and large airway obstruction	↑↑↑	↑↑	↑	More negative	↑↑	↑↑↑
Restrictive lung disease	N	N	N	More negative	↑↑	↑

Lung Oscillometry and Asthma

In small airway disease-asthma (SAD-asthma) and cough variant asthma, even in a background of normal spirometry, lung oscillometry can help in confirmation of diagnosis in this subset of population.

Reduction in R_5 >30% is suggestive of significant post-bronchodilator reversibility.

Reduction in X_5 by 40% and A_x by 50% is also suggestive of significant post-bronchodilator reversibility.

Lung Oscillometry and COPD

In COPD, which is predominantly a disease of smaller airways (R_{5-20}) will be higher compared to a patient with asthma, X_5 will be more negative, and it suggests the severity of dynamic hyperinflation in that patient.

Quality Assurance–Coherence Value and Covariance

In IOS, coherence value is used to determine the validity of results. Coherence value should be between 0.9 and 1.0. Average value of 3–4 signifies technically acceptable recordings which may be considered for calculations.

Covariance commonly used to determine whether a measurement contains too many artefacts between flow and pressure at each frequency, and if it high should be discarded.[25]

Covariance should be used over coherence to determine quality control. Covariance should be <10% in adults and <15% in children for 2 sets of R_5.

A maximum of three acceptable maneuvers are recorded and checked for coherence or covariance.

CONCLUSION

Lung oscillometry is a very useful armamentarium that helps in diagnosis and monitoring the progression of a lung disease by measuring the mechanical properties of lung.

Compared to spirometry, lung oscillometry can detect airway abnormalities at an earlier stage. Regarding asthma, in cough variant asthma and small airway disease-asthma (SAD-asthma), FOT has helped in accurately diagnosing disease in this subset of patients.[26]

The main limitation of FOT/IOS is the lack of reference values and extensive evaluation needed for different disease conditions, which will be addressed as more studies happen in FOT/IOS.

REFERENCES

1. Desai U, Joshi JM. Impulse oscillometry. Adv Respir Med 2019;87(4):235–8.

2. Goldman MD, Saadeh C, Ross D. Clinical applications of forced oscillation to assess peripheral airway function. Respir Physiol Neurobiol 2005;148(1–2):179–94.

3. The forced oscillation technique in clinical practice: methodology, recommendations and future developments | European Respiratory Society [Internet]. [cited 2023 Aug 3];Available from: https://erj.ersjournals.com/content/22/6/1026

4. Brashier B, Salvi S. Measuring lung function using sound waves: role of the forced oscillation technique and impulse oscillometry system. Breathe (Sheff) [Internet] 2015 [cited 2023 Aug 2];11(1):57–65. Available from: https://www.ncbi.nlm.nih.gov/pmc/articles/PMC4487383/

5. Desiraju K, Agrawal A. Impulse oscillometry: The state-of-art for lung function testing. Lung India: Official Organ of Indian Chest Society [Internet] 2016 [cited 2023 Aug 3];33(4):410. Available from: https://www.ncbi.nlm.nih.gov/pmc/articles/PMC4948229/

6. Rasam S, Kodgule R, Vanjare N, Agarwal A, Salvi S. Bronchodilator reversibility using Impulse Oscillometry to differentiate between asthma and COPD. European Respiratory Journal [Internet] 2017 [cited 2023 Aug 4];50(suppl 61). Available from: https://erj.ersjournals.com/content/50/suppl_61/PA2492

7. Airway reversibility assessed by oscillometry in patients with asthma | European Respiratory Society [Internet]. [cited 2023 Aug 4];Available from: https://erj.ersjournals.com/content/50/suppl_61/PA3582

8. Marotta A, Klinnert MD, Price MR, Larsen GL, Liu AH. Impulse oscillometry provides an effective measure of lung dysfunction in 4-year-old children at risk for persistent asthma. Journal of Allergy and Clinical Immunology [Internet] 2003 [cited 2023 Aug 4];112(2):317–22. Available from: https://www.jacionline.org/article/S0091-6749(03)01558-6/fulltext

9. Oscillometry – The future of estimating pulmonary functions – Karnataka Paediatric Journal [Internet]. [cited 2023 Aug 4];Available from: https://iap-kpj.org/oscillometry-the-future-of-estimating-pulmonary-functions/

10. Translational Physiology: Oscillometry of the respiratory system: a translational opportunity not to be missed – PMC [Internet]. [cited 2023 Aug 4];Available from: https://www.ncbi.nlm.nih.gov/pmc/articles/PMC8203417/

11. de Oliveira Jorge PP, de Lima JHP, Chong E Silva DC, Medeiros D, Solé D, Wandalsen GF. Impulse oscillometry in the assessment of children's lung function. Allergol Immunopathol (Madr) 2019;47(3):295–302.

12. McNulty W, Usmani OS. Techniques of assessing small airways dysfunction. Eur Clin Respir J [Internet] 2014 [cited 2023 Aug 4];1:10.3402/ecrj.v1.25898. Available from: https://www.ncbi.nlm.nih.gov/pmc/articles/PMC4629724/

13. Crim C, Celli B, Edwards LD, Wouters E, Coxson HO, Tal-Singer R, et al. Respiratory system impedance with impulse oscillometry in healthy and COPD subjects: ECLIPSE baseline results. Respiratory Medicine [Internet] 2011 [cited 2023 Aug 4];105(7):1069–78. Available from: https://www.sciencedirect.com/science/article/pii/S0954611111000254

14. Komarow HD, Myles IA, Uzzaman A, Metcalfe DD. Impulse oscillometry in the evaluation of diseases of the airways in children. Ann Allergy Asthma Immunol [Internet] 2011 [cited 2023 Aug 4];106(3):191–9. Available from: https://www.ncbi.nlm.nih.gov/pmc/articles/PMC3401927/

15. Bednarek M, Grabicki M, Piorunek T, Batura-Gabryel H. "Current place of impulse oscillometry in the assessment of pulmonary diseases." Respiratory Medicine [Internet] 2020 [cited 2023 Aug 4];170. Available from: https://www.resmedjournal.com/article/S0954-6111(20)30092-5/fulltext

16. Wawszczak M, Kulus M, Peradzyńska J. Peripheral airways involvement in children with asthma exacerbation. Clin Respir J [Internet] 2021 [cited 2023 Aug 5];16(2):97–104. Available from: https://www.ncbi.nlm.nih.gov/pmc/articles/PMC9060097/

17. Guo YF, Herrmann F, Michel JP, Janssens JP. Normal values for respiratory resistance using forced oscillation in subjects and >65 years old. European Respiratory Journal [Internet] 2005 [cited 2023 Aug 6];26(4):602–8. Available from: https://erj.ersjournals.com/content/26/4/602

18. Chaiwong W, Namwongprom S, Liwsrisakun C, Pothirat C. Diagnostic Ability of Impulse Oscillometry in Diagnosis of Chronic Obstructive Pulmonary Disease. COPD 2020;17(6):635–46.
19. Klitgaard A, Løkke A, Hilberg O. Impulse Oscillometry as a Diagnostic Test for Pulmonary Emphysema in a Clinical Setting. J Clin Med [Internet] 2023 [cited 2023 Aug 6];12(4):1547. Available from: https://www.ncbi.nlm.nih.gov/pmc/articles/PMC9967696/
20. Bickel S, Popler J, Lesnick B, Eid N. Impulse oscillometry: interpretation and practical applications. Chest 2014;146(3):841–7.
21. Gong SG, Yang WL, Zheng W, Liu JM. Evaluation of respiratory impedance in patients with chronic obstructive pulmonary disease by an impulse oscillation system. Mol Med Rep 2014;10(5):2694–700.
22. Liu Z, Lin L, Liu X. Clinical application value of impulse oscillometry in geriatric patients with COPD. Int J Chron Obstruct Pulmon Dis 2017;12:897–905.
23. Lung Function Tests in Infants and Children – PMC [Internet]. [cited 2023 Aug 6];Available from: https://www.ncbi.nlm.nih.gov/pmc/articles/PMC10233185/
24. Komarow HD, Young M, Nelson C, Metcalfe DD. Vocal cord dysfunction as demonstrated by impulse oscillometry. J Allergy Clin Immunol Pract 2013;1(4):387–93.
25. Starczewska-Dymek L, Bożek A, Dymek T. Application of the forced oscillation technique in diagnosing and monitoring asthma in preschool children. Adv Respir Med 2019;87(1):26–35.
26. Oppenheimer BW, Goldring RM, Herberg ME, Hofer IS, Reyfman PA, Liautaud S, et al. Distal airway function in symptomatic subjects with normal spirometry following World Trade Center dust exposure. Chest 2007;132(4):1275–82.

Impulse Oscillometry in Obstructive Airway Diseases

• R Venkateswara Babu

Impulse oscillometry is a novel pulmonary function test which is gaining acceptance in recent times. Whether it is useful in diagnosis and follow-up of obstructive airway diseases has been a matter of debate. In this chapter, let us discuss about the usefulness of impulse oscillometry in obstructive airway diseases especially asthma and COPD.

Before we discuss about the usefulness of impulse oscillometry, it is essential that we understand the basic concepts of the mechanics of sound wave propagation through the airways and get familiarized with the various parameters assessed in IOS.

Whenever a pressure wave is transmitted through the airways, certain forces oppose the impulse. These forces are the resistance and reactance of the airways. Resistance reflects the different resistive properties of the airways. Whereas reactance is due to the viscoelastic and inertive properties of the respiratory tract. The sum of both resistance and reactance is known as the respiratory impedance. Hence, the sum of all the forces which oppose the sound wave impulse is the respiratory impedance (Fig. 7.1).

Now, let us discuss about the individual components that make up the respiratory impedance.

Resistance

In the technique of impulse oscillometry (IOS), sound waves are artificially generated and transmitted through the airways. The effect of these sound waves transmitted through the airways is studied in the IOS technique.

When sound waves travel through the airways, higher frequency sound waves travel only shorter distances. Lower frequency sound waves travel further reaching the smaller airways <2 mm in diameter.

The resistance offered by the airways to higher frequency sound waves especially 20 Hz reflects the resistance in the larger airways. It is represented as R_{20} and is the proximal resistance. The resistance offered

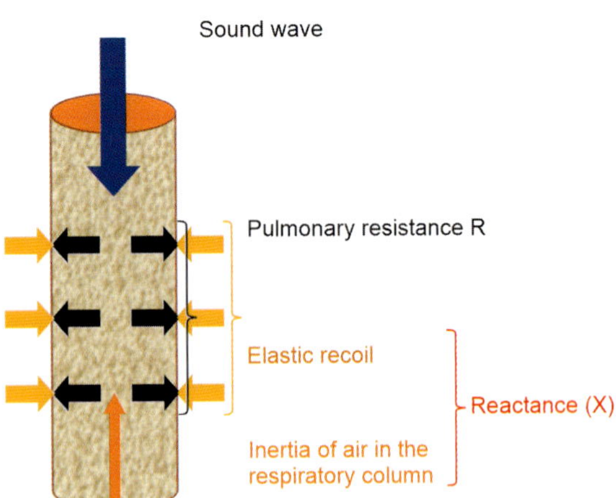

Fig. 7.1: Respiratory impedance is denoted as Z_{rs}, resistance is denoted as R_{rs}, reactance is denoted as X_{rs}, **Respiratory impedance (Z_{rs}) = Respiratory resistance (R_{rs}) + reactance (X_{rs})**

by the airways to lower frequency sound waves, viz. 5 Hz reflects the total lung resistance. It is represented as R_5 (Fig. 7.2). By subtracting R_{20} from R_5 (R_{5-20}), we get the value of the resistance in the small airways.

In a healthy adult, the small airways contribute to a meagre percentage of the resistance since the cross-sectional area is high. Hence, resistance is the same both at 5 Hz and 20 Hz.

The next parameter that contributes to the impedance is the reactance of the respiratory tract.

Reactance

The reactance of the airways is contributed by 2 factors: Capacitance and inertance.

When sound waves travel through the airways, the elasticity of the airways opposes the sound impulses. The elasticity of the airways is mainly contributed by the small airways. This is known as '**capacitance (C)**'. Usually, capacitance effects are reported as negative numbers (Fig. 7.3).

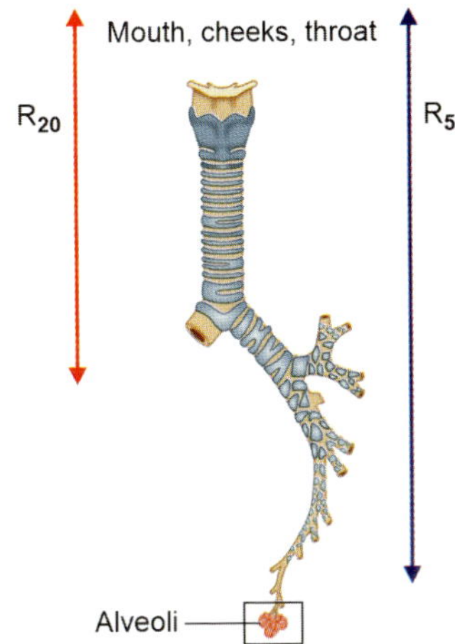

Fig. 7.2: Distances travelled by sound waves of different frequencies: R_5—total lung resistance; R_{20}—proximal resistance; R_{5-20}—resistance in the small airways (*Adapted from [1]*)

When sound waves travel through the airways, the other factor that opposes the sound impulses is the inertial property of the airways. The inertial effect is mainly due to the larger airways. This is known as '**inertance (I)**'. Inertance effects are reported as positive numbers (Fig. 7.3).

Reactance is the sum total of capacitance and inertance.

$$Reactance\ (X_{rs}) = Capacitance\ (C) + Inertance\ (I)$$

[Typically, the reactance is measured at 5 Hz (X_5)].

At low frequencies (between 2 and 10 Hz) capacitance effects predominate. At high frequencies (between 10 and 30 Hz) inertance effects predominate. Hence, reactance actually reflects the balance between inertial and elastic properties of the airways.

Having understood resistance and reactance, it is important that we are familiar with two other parameters which are useful in the interpretation of impulse oscillometry—the resonant frequency and reactance area.

Resonant Frequency

At a particular frequency, the inertial and capacitance components balance and cancel each other out. This is known as the '**resonant frequency**—indicated by F_{res}. **Normal F_{res} is approximately 7–12 Hz** (Figs 7.3 and 7.4). The resonant frequency decreases with age. In obstructive airway disorders, the resonant frequency increases.

Reactance Area

It is the area bounded by a line at 5 Hz up to the resonant frequency F_{res}. This is a measure of the frequencies wherein capacitance dominates over inertance. It is indicated by A_x and is also called the **Goldman triangle** (Fig. 7.3).

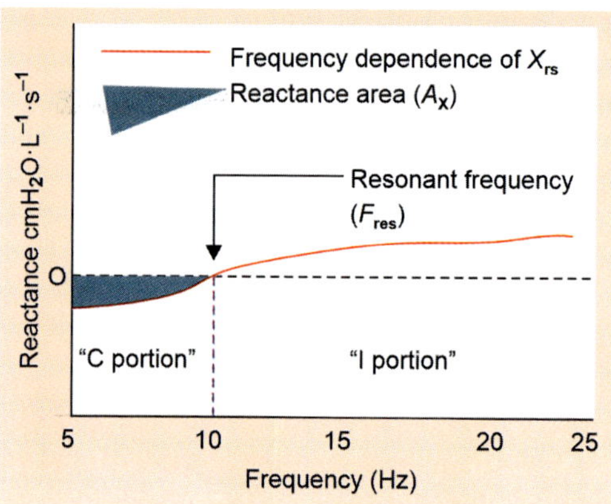

Fig. 7.3: Reactance values in a healthy adult. C—compliance and I—inertance portions of reactance; F_{res}—resonant frequency; A_x—area of reactance (*Adapted from [1]*)

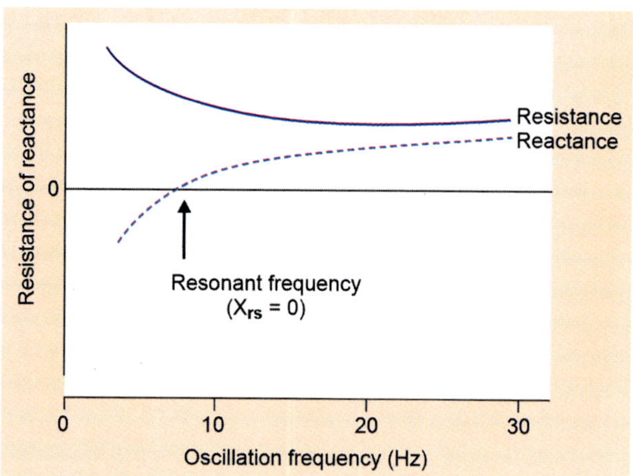

Fig. 7.4: Frequency dependence of resistance and of reactance. Resonant frequency is the frequency at which reactance (X_{rs}) is 0 (*Adapted from [2]*)

The normal values of the various oscillometric parameters as seen in a normal healthy adult is summarized below.

Parameter	Normal healthy adult
R_5	Normal
R_{20}	Normal
R_{5-20}	Close to zero
X_5	Normal
A_x	Normal
Resonant frequency	7–12 Hz

R_5: Airway resistance at 5 Hz, R_{20}: Airway resistance at 20 Hz, X_5: Respiratory reactance at 5 Hz, A_x: Reactance area

OSCILLOMETRIC CHANGES IN OBSTRUCTIVE AIRWAY DISEASES

Resistance

In cases of airway obstruction, R_5 is increased above normal. When there is large airway obstruction, the airway resistance elevates evenly. When there is small/peripheral airways obstruction, the resistance increases at low frequencies, and then starts decreasing as the frequency increases (Fig. 7.5). So, the resistance is frequency dependent.

Reactance

In obstructive airway diseases like asthma and COPD, the respiratory system becomes less compliant and becomes stiffer. So, the reactance becomes more negative. Resultantly, the reactance area (A_x) increases and the F_{res} increases (Fig. 7.6).

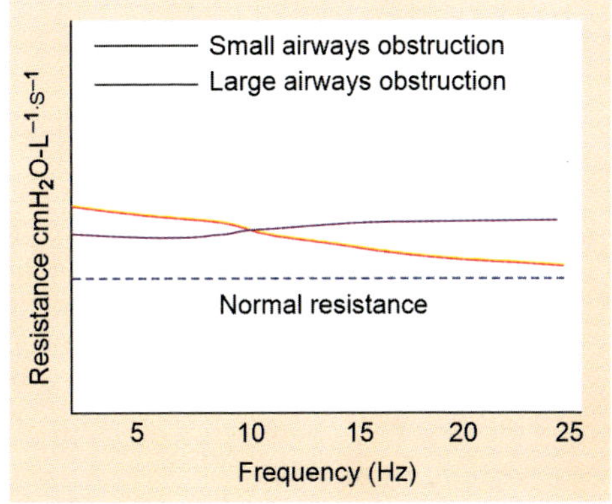

Fig. 7.5: Changes in resistance in small airway obstruction and large airway obstruction *(Adapted from [1])*

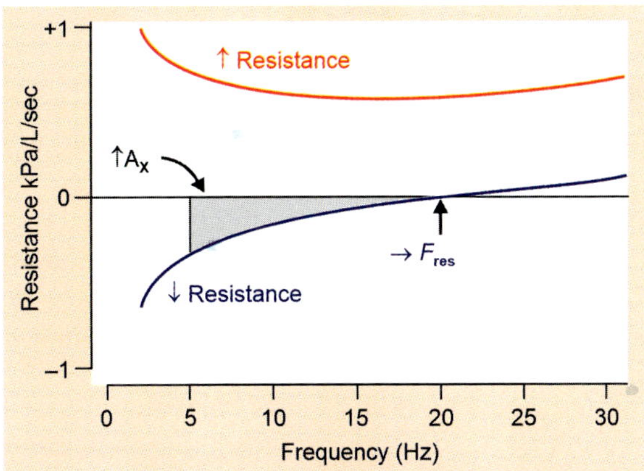

Fig. 7.6: Changes in oscillometric parameters in obstructive airway diseases

The effects of obstructive airway diseases on the various oscillometric parameters, as compared to a normal healthy adult is summarised below.

Parameter	Normal healthy adult	Central airway obstruction	Peripheral airway obstruction with alveolar damage
R_5	Normal	>150% predicted	>150% predicted
R_{20}	Normal	>150% predicted	Normal
R_{5-20}	Close to zero	Close to zero	Increased
X_5	Normal	Normal	Increased
A_x	Normal	Normal	Increased
Resonant frequency (F_{res})	7–12 Hz	Normal	Increased

R_5: Airway resistance at 5 Hz, R_{20}: Airway resistance at 20 Hz, X_5: Respiratory reactance at 5 Hz, A_x: Reactance area

CRITERIA FOR BRONCHODILATOR RESPONSE IN IMPULSE OSCILLOMETRY IN ADULTS

In 2020, the European Respiratory Journal had published the technical standards for impulse oscillometry.[2] According to the standards, the thresholds for defining a positive bronchodilator response are:

- 50% increase in X_{rs5}
- 40% decrease in R_{rs5}, and
- 80% decrease in A_x

BRONCHIAL CHALLENGE TESTING

When bronchial challenge testing is done using impulse oscillometry, there is increased sensitivity of detecting bronchoconstriction.[2] Hence, the total dose required would be less.

But it is very difficult to assess airway hyper-responsiveness (AHR) based on oscillometry. Many studies have been done to define the threshold wherein the results vary widely. The results range from a 20 to 50% increase in R_5 and a 20–80% decrease in X_5.

ASTHMA VS COPD BY IMPULSE OSCILLOMETRY

In bronchial asthma, the change in both resistance and reactance is usually in a proportionate fashion. Whereas in COPD, resistance usually alters to a relatively lesser degree compared to reactance.

CLINICAL APPLICATION OF IMPULSE OSCILLOMETRY IN COPD

According to global initiative for obstructive lung disease (GOLD), the diagnostic criteria for COPD is a post-bronchodilator FEV_1/VC ratio <0.7.

An editorial in European Respiratory Journal in 2023 states that by the time we are able to diagnose airflow obstruction by the above-mentioned criteria by spirometry, patients have lost a significant proportion (at least 40%) of their terminal bronchioles.[3] So, the diagnosis is quite delayed by spirometry. In such cases when spirometry is normal, impulse oscillometry would be able to pick up early small airway disease.[4,5]

In the review article by Kaminsky et al,[6] it has been stated that IOS would be able to pick up early the adverse effects of smoking before COPD is diagnosed. It has been shown by various studies that there is a high prevalence of abnormal impedance in smokers with normal spirometry mainly in the R_{rs} and X_{rs} near 5 Hz.[7–10]

In the review article by Lipworth and Jabbal,[11] it has been stated that both R_{5-20} and A_x are closely related to COPD severity and exacerbations. Both the parameters significantly improve after administration of long-acting bronchodilators. In COPD, since there is absence of large airway involvement, R_{20} does not improve with bronchodilatation or bronchoconstriction. In future, we have to do more studies to see if impulse oscillometry can be combined with spirometry to predict future exacerbations. It is also postulated that A_x might be useful as a screening tool in early-stage of COPD.

In COPD patients, Gong et al have shown that changes in X_5 over time might be used for monitoring the disease progression.[12]

CLINICAL APPLICATION OF IMPULSE OSCILLOMETRY IN ASTHMA

In the review article by Kaminsky et al,[6] it has been stated that in bronchial asthma patients, even when spirometry is normal, impulse oscillometry would be able to pick up airway obstruction. Also, when compared to spirometry IOS would have a higher sensitivity in assessing response to bronchodilators.

In patients of bronchial asthma, small airway dysfunction (SAD) can be present even in the absence of symptoms and normal spirometry. SAD is an early sign in the pathogenesis of asthma. To assess the extent of SAD in asthma, the multinational ATLANTIS (Assessment of small Airways Involvement in Asthma) study was conducted.[13] ATLANTIS tried to find out which combination of biomarkers, physiological test and imaging markers best measured SAD in asthma patients. The results of the large ATLANTIS study revealed that the IOS parameters R_{rs5-20}, A_x and X_{rs5} were all strong contributors to SAD and thus play an important role in identifying SAD in asthma.[14]

Foy and colleagues provided direct evidence on how R_{5-20} reflects airway narrowing in specific locations of the bronchial tree. This strengthens the concept that R_{5-20} is a useful tool to measure small airway disease in asthma.[15]

LIMITATIONS OF IMPULSE OSCILLOMETRY IN OBSTRUCTIVE AIRWAY DISEASES

The predictive equations for IOS parameters are very few worldwide. It is quite difficult to apply the existing reference equations across different devices and different manufacturers. In order to validate the available data, we have to conduct more studies worldwide in different geographical regions of the world. Only then it is possible to get valid global references of the parameters. Also, there is no data on the grading of severity of airway obstruction.

CONCLUSION

Spirometry is an effort dependent procedure. In contrast, oscillometry test outcomes can be derived from tidal breathing. Hence, there is less room for errors.

Impulse oscillometry is a very simple test to perform in our outpatient department. But the interpretation remains a huge challenge. It is a better tool for identifying and measurement of small airway dysfunction (SAD), early diagnosis of COPD in smokers and to predict asthma control and exacerbations. However, due to the lack of multi-ethnic population normal values across all ages, large clinical studies are required before this promising tool becomes a routine clinical investigation.

REFERENCES

1. Bill Brashier, Sundeep Salvi. Measuring lung function using sound waves: role of the forced oscillation technique and impulse oscillometry system. Breathe 2015;11:1.

2. King GG, Bates J, Berger KI, et al. Technical standards for respiratory oscillometry. Eur Respir J 2020;55: 1900753.

3. Ananth S, Hurst JR. ERJ advances: state of the art in definitions and diagnosis of COPD. Eur Respir J 2023;61:2202318

4. Desai U, Joshi JM. Impulse oscillometry. Adv Respir Med 2019;87:235–38.

5. Xu J, Sun X, Zhu H, et al. Long-term variability of impulse oscillometry and spirometry in stable COPD and asthma. Respir Res 2022;23:262.

6. Kaminsky DA, Simpson SJ, Berger KI, et al. Clinical significance and applications of oscillometry. Eur Respir Rev 2022;31:210208.

7. Faria AC, Costa AA, Lopes AJ, et al. Forced oscillation technique in the detection of smoking-induced respiratory alterations: diagnostic accuracy and comparison with spirometry. Clinics 2010;(96)65: 1295–1304.

8. Faria AC, Lopes AJ, Jansen JM, et al. Evaluating the forced oscillation technique in the detection of early smoking-induced respiratory changes. Biomed Eng 2009;8:22.

9. Jetmalani K, Thamrin C, Farah CS, et al. Peripheral airway dysfunction and relationship with symptoms in smokers with preserved spirometry. Respirology 2017;23:512–18.

10. Shinke H, Yamamoto M, Hazeki N, et al. Visualized changes in respiratory resistance and reactance along a time axis in smokers: a cross-sectional study. Respir Investig 2013;51:166–74.

11. Brian J. Lipworth, Sunny Jabbal. What can we learn about COPD from impulse oscillometry. Respiratory Medicine 2018;139:106–109.

12. Gong SG, Yang WL, Zheng W, Liu JM. Evaluation of respiratory impedance in patients with chronic obstructive pulmonary disease by an impulse oscillation system. Mol Med Rep 2014;10:2694–700.

13. Postma DS, Brightling C, Baldi S, Van den Berge M, Fabbri LM, Gagnatelli A, et al. Exploring the relevance and extent of small airways dysfunction in asthma (ATLANTIS): baseline data from a prospective cohort study. Lancet Respir Med. 2019;7:402–16.

14. Kraft M, Richardson M, Hallmark B, et al. The role of small airways dysfunction in asthma control and exacerbations: a longitudinal, observational analysis using data from the ATLANTIS study. Lancet Respir Med 2022;20:661–68.

15. Foy BH, Soares M, Bordas R, Richardson M, Bell A, Singapuri A, et al. Lung computational models and the role of the small airways in asthma. Am J Respir Crit Care Med 2019;200:982–91.

Oscillometry in Restrictive Airway Diseases

• Daksh Sharma

Impulse oscillometry (IOS) is a non-invasive method that only necessitates the patient's passive engagement to measure respiratory impedance.[1] It is capable of evaluating two respiratory impedance variables: Respiratory resistance and reactance. Total airway resistance is represented by the 5 Hz (R_5) resistance at low frequency, while central airway resistance is roughly represented by the 20 Hz (R_{20}) resistance at high frequency. IOS is based on forced oscillation technique (FOT) which uses sound waves of different frequencies in interpretation and takes longer time compared to IOS. There are machines based on FOT and IOS and different facilities use them in accordance with their conveniences.

The variance between R_5 and R_{20} (R_{5-20}) serves as a measure of the small airways.[2] Compliance and reactance at 5 Hz (X_5) are believed to be inversely related. Reactance area (A_x) is the integrated low frequency respiratory reactance magnitude (area under the curve) between 5 Hz and resonant frequency (F_{res}), where resonant frequency (F_{res}) is the intermediate frequency at which the total reactance is 0. X_5, F_{res}, and A_x are been recommended for detecting expiratory flow limitations. IOS accurately identify elevated airway resistance both in small and central airways, hence it has been utilized mostly for patients with obstructive lung disorders like COPD and bronchial asthma.

Interstitial lung diseases modify the lung's mechanical and gas exchange characteristics. Typically, interstitial lung diseases are characterized by restrictive changes in pulmonary physiology, including decreased diffusing capacity for carbon monoxide (DLCO), decreased residual volume, decreased static compliance and a reduced VC.[3]

ILDs are also associated with small airway dysfunction therefore, several authors have tried to explain the utility of IOS in various forms of ILDs. Some of them have concluded that, a lower X_5 is indicative of a restricted pattern patients with ILD, X_5 and FEV_1/FVC have an inverse relationship.[3] This chapter will be dealing with various ILDs and their characteristic IOS findings.

HYPERSENSITIVITY PNEUMONITIS (HP)

HP or extrinsic allergic alevolitis is a condition that is brought on by an abnormal immune lung response to diverse inhaled antigens and abnormal lung immunological reaction to an array of inhaled antigens.[4] Most cases of HP are caused by antigens associated frequent contact with house ornamental birds kept inside homes. Patients with HP exhibit small airway involvement on their lung biopsy specimens. The pathological manifestations of small airway (SA) involvement include, ill formed non-necrotizing granulomas, interstitium is filled by mononuclear cells and various extent of fibrosis.[5]

Selene Guerrero Zúñiga et al, did an analysis to determine the small airway function in the patients of hypersensitivity pneumonitis by IOS and they found that all the patients had high A_x; 40% elevated R_5, R_{5-20}; 100% low X_5.[6] In another study the authors designed to measure small airway resistance (R_{5-20}), resistance (R_5), and reactance (X_5) on inspiration, expiration, and post-bronchodilator response by forced oscillation technique (FOT), in 28 subjects suffering from hypersensitivity pneumonitis. Pre- and post-bronchodilator PFTs with plethysmography, lung carbon monoxide diffusing capacity (DLCO), and FOT measures were done, they concluded that the only three (8%) of the patients showed elevated R_5 values. Moreover, all subjects had low X_5 values, which indicated poorer lung compliance and R_5, X_5, and R_{5-19} data revealed no bronchodilator response in any subjects.[5]

SARCOIDOSIS

Sarcoidosis is an inflammatory condition, where the granulomas are the hallmark of this disease, which can occur in virtually any organ.[7] Clinical and radiological diversity is a prominent feature of pulmonary sarcoidosis and respiratory impairments coupled with increased airway obstruction and decreased pulmonary compliance.[8] Spirometry and other pulmonary function tests like body plethysmography and DLCO are typically used to assess the respiratory variations in these patients with sarcoidosis and these tests demand great effort, it requires coordinated efforts from the patients during both inhalations and exhalations. Hence, patients with advance disease would ought to avoid it.[9,10]

Therefore, IOS could be a novel alternative to pulmonary function tests to access the small airway function in patients with sarcoidosis on the grounds that IOS measures central and peripheral lung mechanical characteristics by superimposing pressure variations over tidal breathing. Low frequency (5 Hz) measurements might reveal alterations in the small airways.[11]

Consequently, E. Renzoni et al investigated IOS characteristics in 63 pulmonary sarcoidosis patients prospectively, and identified relationships with respiratory symptoms and traditional lung function tests. They found increased A_x, F_{res}, and more negative (decreased) X_5 which is consistent with a restrictive pattern. They also concluded that, there was a strong correlation between IOS outcomes R_5, X_5, F_{res}, A_x, but not R_{20}, and lung volumes (FEV$_1$%, FVC%, RV/TLV), as well as maximal expiratory flows (MEF 75%, MEF 50%, MEF 25%). In addition, there was a strong correlation between the R_5, X_5, F_{res}, and A_x values and the overall SGRQ scores (rho = 0.41, –0.43, 0.38, and 0.44, respectively; p <0.01).

SCLERODERMA ILD

Systemic sclerosis (SSc) is a diverse illness with an uncertain etiology, it is characterized by autoimmunity, vasculopathy, fibrosis and a few available therapeutic options.[12] SSc can cause severe complications, including ILD, which is a common and early consequence of this disease, it has been linked to substantial morbidity and mortality. SSc-ILD severity is now determined through spirometery DLCO and body plethysmography along with lung high-resolution computed tomography (HRCT) analysis.[13]

IOS offers a non-invasive less cumbersome approach for assessment of lung mechanics in such patients. However, IOS is not been extensively investigated in SCC patients. In a study, David Aronsson and colleagues determined the IOS characteristics of patients with SCC and compared it with 28 non-smoking normal subjects. They enrolled 88 patients in total out of which 65 patients had limited disease and 13 had diffuse disease. The authors concluded that when measured by IOS, the group of limited SSc patients showed a markedly higher level of resistance and reactance (such as A_x and F_{res}) than the healthy controls, patients with diffuse SSc did not display an increase in IOS parameters, the potential cause of resistance and reactance measurements by IOS being indicative of initial alterations in essiential lung inflammation in SSc patients.[14]

In conclusion, SSc patients have increased reactance and resistance in their small airways. The positive relationship between airway reactance and ground-glass opacity may indicate that altered parameters of IOS may represent early diseases.[14]

IDIOPATHIC PULMONARY FIBROSIS

Idiopathic pulmonary fibrosis (IPF) is a chronic, advancing disease that affects the lungs' parenchyma and is marked by an unusual proliferation of fibrotic tissue. It has a high mortality rate and a dismal prognosis.[15] The vital capacity (VC), forced vital capacity (FVC), and diffusing lung capacity for carbon monoxide (DLCO) variables of the pulmonary function test (PFT) have been linked to prognosis in individuals with IPF.

Apart from increased extracellular matrix deposition in the lung interstitium scarring along with fibrosis are another pathogenic aspect of IPF is small airway dysfunction associated with terminal bronchiole loss.[16] In IPF patients, the identification of small airway abnormalities can also direct the use of bronchodilators among symptomatic patients.[17,18] Verleden et al utilized multi-detector CT, micro-CT, and histology to assess IPF patients, they concluded that small airway illness has been believed to be a part of IPF and a potential treatment target for the condition.[19]

When it comes to identifying small airway dysfunction, IOS is much more precise than spirometry. Most patients of IPF have advanced disease which make them unfit for performing various effort-dependent PFTs due to underlying breathlessness. Hence, it is favorable in patients who cannot execute effort-dependent exhalation due to shortness of breath and severe coughing.[20]

To ascertain the effectiveness of FOT in IPF patients, Yuki Mori et al included 97 cases of IPF. Authors also tried to establish the relationship between the FOT, percentage forced vital capacity (FVC), vital capacity (VC), forced expiratory volume in 1 second (FEV_1). The authors came to a conclusion that the, R_5 (whole breath, Ex, In); R_{20} (whole breath, Ex, In); R_{5-20} (whole breath, In) and A_x were inversely correlated with VC, FEV_1, FVC. Furthermore, the X_5 was strongly linked with these values (r = 0.5–0.6, p <0.01).[21]

RHEUMATOID ARTHRITIS (RA) ASSOCIATED INTERSTITIAL LUNG DISEASE

RA manifests differently depending on the stage of the disease and has a substantial influence on most body organs in addition to the joints.[22] Up to 60% of RA patients may experience lung involvement during the advancement of the illness, which makes it the most prevalent extra-articular expression of the disease.[23] The involvement of the lungs, particularly RA-ILD, is linked to substantial morbidity and mortality.[24] Patients with RA have an airway disease prevalence of 39–60%, and both large as well as small airways could be affected.[25] It is difficult to analyse small airways independently. Spirometry has been the method most utilised for determining the severity of small airway illness, although it has drawbacks.

Hence, Reham M and colleagues investigated the utility of FOT in sixty RA-ILD patients. They made 2 groups, first being the RA patients with normal spirometry group and the second one being the RA patients with abnormal spirometry group, both had 26 and 34 patients respectively. Lung resistance at Hz (R_{20}), 5 Hz (R_5), i.e. central airway resistance, total airway resistance respectively and area of reactance (A_x) was greater in these subjects and reactance at 5 Hz (X_5) was curtailed.[26]

Conversely, though Wen-Chien Cheng et al found that the R_5, R_{5-20}, F_{res} were increased and A_x was reduced in RA cases with abnormal lung CT scans. Both the studies show that there is both central and peripheral lung involvement in RA.

CONCLUSION

Considering that certain researchers have discovered combination of central and peripheral airways involvement while others have discovered a typical restrictive pattern, the IOS characteristics in different types of ILD varies. The pathognomonic feature of ILD on IOS is therefore very difficult to mention. As the data on IOS and ILD is sparse, it might be challenging to analyse resistance and reactance curves, need expertise and experience, which is one of the main constraints. In a broader sense, IOS can be utilized as an adjunctive test alongside other PFT in the diagnosis and follow-up of restrictive lung diseases because it is non-invasive, less labour-intensive and can even be performed at patient's bedside.

REFERENCES

1. Sugiyama A, Hattori N, Haruta Y, Nakamura I, et al. Characteristics of inspiratory and expiratory reactance in interstitial lung disease. Respir Med 2013;107(6):875–82.
2. Kubota M, Shirai G, Nakamori T, et al. Low frequency oscillometry parameters in COPD patients are less variable during inspiration than during expiration. Respir Physiol Neurobiol 2009;166(2):73–9.
3. Naglaa BA, Kamal E et al. Role of IOS in evaluation of patients with interstitial lung diseases. Egyptian Journal of Chest Diseases and Tuberculosis 2016;65(4):791–5.
4. Lacasse Y, Girard M, Cormier Y et al. Recent advances in hypersensitivity pneumonitis. Chest 2012;142(1):208–17.
5. Gaxiola M, Buendía-Roldán I, Mejía M, et al. Morphologic diversity of chronic pigeon breeder's disease: clinical features and survival. Respir Med 2011;105(4):608–14.
6. Guerrero Zúñiga S, Sánchez Hernández J, Mateos Toledo, et al. Small airway dysfunction in chronic hypersensitivity pneumonitis. Respirology 2017;22(8):1637–42.
7. Sarcoidosis | Nature Reviews Disease Primers [Internet]. [cited 2023 Aug 4];Available from: https://www.nature.com/articles/s41572-019-0096-x
8. Brådvik I, Wollmer P, Simonsson B, Albrechtsson U, et al. Lung mechanics and their relationship to lung volumes in pulmonary sarcoidosis. Eur Respir J 1989;2(7):643–51.
9. Explainable machine learning methods and respiratory oscillometry for the diagnosis of respiratory abnormalities in sarcoidosis | BMC Medical Informatics and Decision Making | Full Text [Internet]. [cited 2023 Aug 4];Available from: https://bmcmedinformdecismak.biomedcentral.com/articles/10.1186/s12911-022-02021-2
10. Johannessen A, Lehmann S, Omenaas ER, et al. Post-bronchodilator spirometry reference values in adults and implications for disease management. Am J Respir Crit Care Med 2006;173(12):1316–25.
11. Impulse oscillometry measurements are correlated to quality of life in patients with pulmonary sarcoidosis [Internet]. [cited 2023 Aug 4];Available from: https://www.ers-education.org/lr/show-details/?idP=133468
12. Schoenfeld SR, Castelino FV. Interstitial Lung Disease in Scleroderma. Rheum Dis Clin North Am 2015;41(2):237–48.
13. Matucci-Cerinic M, D'Angelo S, Denton CP, et al. Assessment of lung involvement. Clin Exp Rheumatol 2003;21(3 Suppl 29):S19–23.
14. Aronsson D, Hesselstrand R, Bozovic G, Wuttge DM, et al.. Airway resistance and reactance are affected in systemic sclerosis. Eur Clin Respir J 2015;2:10.3402/ecrj.v2.28667.

15. Sgalla G, Iovene B, Calvello M, Ori M, et al. Idiopathic pulmonary fibrosis: pathogenesis and management. Respiratory Research 2018;19(1):32.

16. Krishna R, Chapman K, Ullah S. Idiopathic Pulmonary Fibrosis [Internet]. In: StatPearls. Treasure Island (FL): StatPearls Publishing; 2023 [cited 2023 Aug 4]. Available from: http://www.ncbi.nlm.nih.gov/books/NBK448162/

17. Hu PW, Ko HK, Su KC, Feng JY, et al. Functional parameters of small airways can guide bronchodilator use in idiopathic pulmonary fibrosis. Sci Rep 2020;10:18633.

18. Verleden SE, Tanabe N, McDonough JE, et al. Small airways pathology in Idiopathic Pulmonary Fibrosis: A retrospective cohort study. Lancet Respir Med 2020;8(6):573–84.

19. Tanabe N, McDonough JE, Vasilescu DM, et al. Pathology of Idiopathic Pulmonary Fibrosis Assessed by a Combination of Microcomputed Tomography, Histology, and Immunohistochemistry. The *American Journal of Pathology* 2020;190(12):2427–35.

20. "Current place of impulse oscillometry in the assessment of pulmonary diseases." – PubMed [Internet]. [cited 2023 Aug 4];Available from: https://pubmed.ncbi.nlm.nih.gov/32843158/

21. Mori Y, Nishikiori H, Chiba H, Yamada G, et al. Respiratory reactance in forced oscillation technique reflects disease stage and predicts lung physiology deterioration in idiopathic pulmonary fibrosis. Respir Physiol Neurobiol 2020;275:103386.

22. Dougados M, Soubrier M, Antunez A, et al. Prevalence of comorbidities in rheumatoid arthritis and evaluation of their monitoring: results of an international, cross-sectional study (COMORA). Ann Rheum Dis 2014;73(1):62–8.

23. Norton S, Koduri G, Nikiphorou E, et al. A study of baseline prevalence and cumulative incidence of comorbidity and extra-articular manifestations in RA and their impact on outcome. Rheumatology (Oxford) 2013;52(1):99–110.

24. Kadura S, Raghu G. Rheumatoid arthritis-interstitial lung disease: manifestations and current concepts in pathogenesis and management. European Respiratory Review [Internet] 2021 [cited 2023 Aug 6];30(160). Available from: https://err.ersjournals.com/content/30/160/210011

25. Singh R, Krishnamurthy P, Deepak D, et al. Small airway disease and its predictors in patients with rheumatoid arthritis. Respiratory Investigation 2022;60(3):379–84.

26. Impulse oscillometry, an aid or a substitute? | The Egyptian Journal of Bronchology Available from: https://ejb.springeropen.com/articles/10.4103/ejb.ejb_98_18

Oscillometry in Large Airway Obstruction

• Muniza Bai

UPPER AIRWAY OBSTRUCTION

The upper airway refers to the portion of the respiratory tract located above the trachea and includes several anatomical structures that play significant roles in breathing and speech. These structures include the nasal cavity, nasopharynx, and larynx. Oscillometry has emerged as a valuable diagnostic tool in the assessment and aids with the management of upper airway obstruction. It offers a non-invasive and comprehensive means of evaluating respiratory function. Upper airway obstruction can result from a myriad of conditions including anatomical abnormalities extending anywhere from nose to epiglottis, inflammatory disorders or neuromuscular dysfunction. Oscillometry has been studied for the assessment of upper airway function during sleep and vocal cord dysfunction.[1–3] However, not many studies are available that have described the role of oscillometry in other causes of upper airway obstruction in adults like chronic rhinosinusitis, laryngeal stenosis or foreign body aspiration. In this chapter, we shall deal with role of oscillometry in airway assessment during sleep and vocal cord dysfunction.

Role of Oscillometry in Upper Airway Obstruction during Sleep

Oscillometry is a non-invasive method to measure the mechanical impedance of the respiratory system. In recent times, it has been studied in sleep disordered breathing, where it measures the variations in the upper airway resistance. Here, small pressure oscillations generated by a loudspeaker, or a continuous positive airway pressure (CPAP) device are superimposed on the nasal pressure when the patient is breathing spontaneously. Flow signals are recorded at the nasal mask and the respiratory impedance is computed from the pressure.

The role of oscillometry in sleep includes:

1. **Assessment of upper airway function:** It provides insights into upper airway mechanics by analysing impedance of the respiratory system. This is based on the collapsibility of the upper airways, which is a major key factor in OSA.
2. **Airway resistance measurement:** The oscillometry technique helps quantify upper airway resistance, aiding in diagnosis and treatment planning.
3. **CPAP titration:** Oscillometry helps with CPAP titration. At CPAP pressures that abolish apneas and hypopneas, FOT signals show low impedance.[4–6]
4. **Treatment monitoring:** After OSA treatment, oscillometry can be used to assess the effectiveness of interventions like CPAP therapy and surgical interventions. Changes in airway resistance and its function can be tracked over time to evaluate treatment outcomes.

5. **Differentiating types of sleep apnea:** Oscillometry can distinguish between central sleep apnea and obstructive sleep apnea. Central sleep apnea is characterized by a lack of effort to breathe, while OSA involves airway obstruction.
6. **Pediatric OSA:** Oscillometry is particularly useful in the pediatric population where polysomnographic studies can be challenging.
7. **Research and study:** It helps in enhanced comprehension of the physiological mechanisms underlying OSA and to develop new diagnostic and treatment approaches.

OSCILLOMETRY IN OBESITY

Thoracic and abdominal adipose tissue accumulation causes reduced compliance of the respiratory system. Reduced expiratory reserve volume and functional residual capacity bring about a decrease in the lung elastic recoil pressure. There is heterogenous airway narrowing and airway closure in the lung peripheries. Due to these factors, individuals with obesity typically show higher peripheral airway resistance and a more negative reactance (X_5) as shown in Fig. 9.1B.[7] These parameters have shown to be moderately closely correlated with OSA severity measured by respiratory disturbance index.[8]

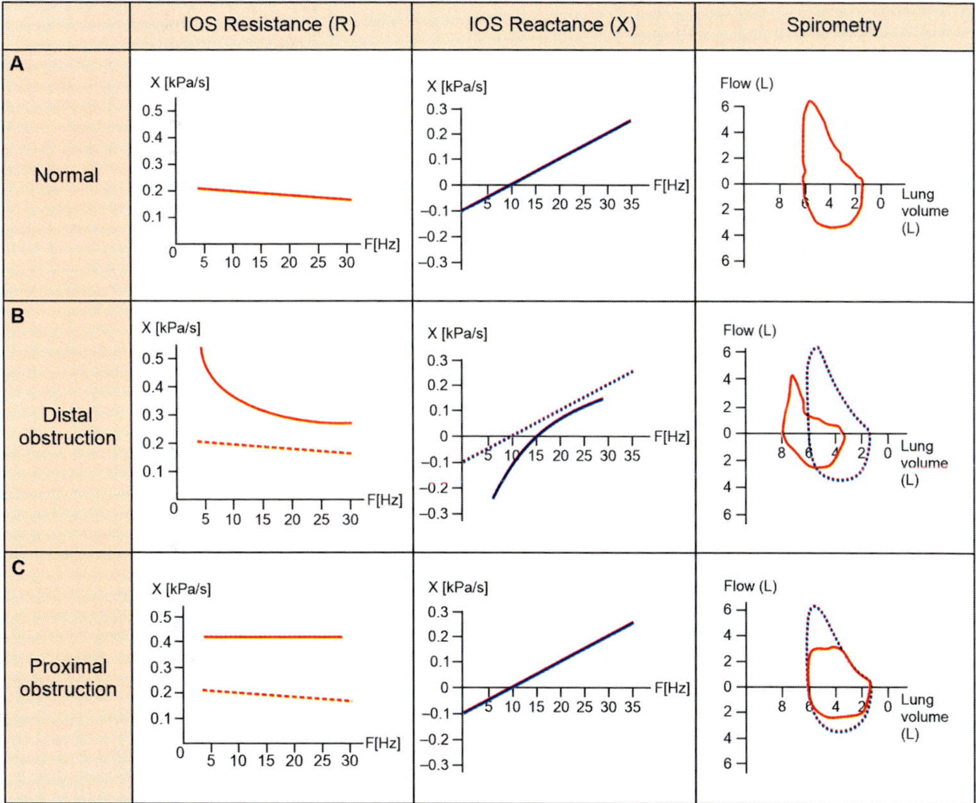

Fig. 9.1: Representative graphs of IOS and spirometry in patients with normal and obstructive airway disease. Tracings of lung resistance (R) and reactance (X) in comparison with spirometric flow-volume loop for patients with normal lung function (A), distal obstruction (B) and proximal obstruction (C). Dotted lines indicate the normal tracing, whereas solid lines indicate pathological tracings

Obese individuals with asthma tend to have a more negative airway reactance than obese non-asthmatic individuals, likely due to increased peripheral airway closure.[9] Oscillometry also provides information on how sleep apnea and bronchial asthma interact to increase airway obstruction.[10] Creation of exaggerated negative intrathoracic pressures against the occluded pharynx during obstructive apneas causes cephalad shift of fluid into the thorax, thereby increasing the intrathoracic fluid which narrows the small airways and increase the airflow resistance. The effect due to cephalad shift of fluid is more marked in bronchial asthma as the small airways have narrow calibre to begin with, making them more susceptible to fluid accumulation around them.

The response to methacholine bronchial challenge test in obese subjects differ when compared to non-obese subjects, with exaggerated decrease in airway reactance. These subtle differences are not seen with spirometry, where typically no changes are seen in case of severe obesity (BMI >40 kg/m^2).[11]

OSCILLOMETRY PARAMETERS IN OBSTRUCTIVE SLEEP APNEA

Below are the oscillometry findings in a case of obstructive sleep apnea due to obesity.
1. Resistance at 5 Hz, R_5 increases
2. Resistance at 20 Hz, R_{20} increases
3. R_{5-20} increases
4. Reactance at 5 Hz, X_5 becomes more negative
5. F_{res} increases
6. Area under the curve, A_x increases

Parameters of oscillometry in obstructive sleep apnea with only upper airway pathology (as shown in Fig. 9.1C) are as follows:
1. Resistance at 5 Hz, R_5 increases
2. Resistance at 20 Hz, R_{20} increases
3. R_{5-20} remains normal
4. Reactance at 5 Hz, X_5 remains normal
5. Area under the curve, A_x remains normal

Common Problems Faced while Using Oscillometry during Sleep

Several problems have been reported in the literature that may affect the impedance values, the most common being leaks.[3] Leaks are a common occurrence during the application of CPAP. Leaks via the mask or the mouth can cause falsely low impedance values. This can be taken care of by analysing the flow signals and interpreting the impedance data along with other information from the sleep recording and not alone. Mouth breathing is another possible problem. Humans usually breathe through the nose; however, it is not uncommon for man to inhale through the nose and exhale through the mouth. During mouth expiration, the soft palate rises and occludes the posterior nares, thereby causing a false increase in impedance. Similarly, there occurs false rise in impedance during wake periods or arousals due to change in the route of breathing (Fig. 9.2). These possible misinterpretations of oscillometry data can be avoided if the flow signal is taken into consideration while interpreting data.

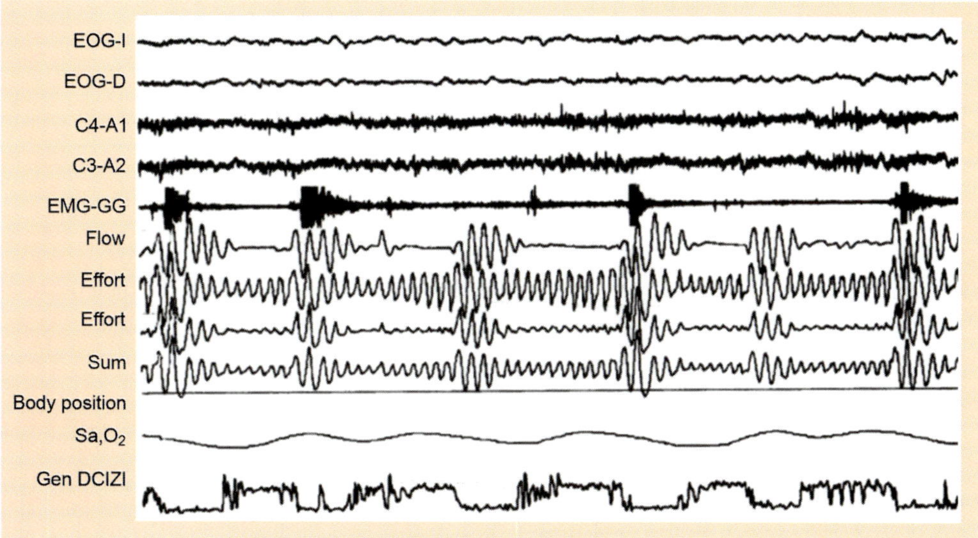

Fig. 9.2: Representative polysomnographic recording with oscillatory impedance at the bottom. Impedance signals show low values during arousals and higher values during periods of apnea–hypopnea

Practical Application of Oscillometry during Sleep

It is not advisable to use oscillometry techniques routinely in all sleep studies. It should be employed in only select population of OSAHS patients in assessing upper airway obstruction, studying upper airway mechanics in various airway events or entities such as Cheyne Stokes respiration. It can be used for CPAP titration and monitoring treatment outcomes.[12]

Though oscillometry can provide valuable insights in sleep studies, it is often used in conjunction with other diagnostic tools and clinical assessments to form a thorough understanding and impression of patient condition. It is important to bear in mind that oscillometry has not been incorporated in the diagnostic armamentarium of sleep related breathing disorders in American Academy of Sleep Medicine guidelines for diagnostics of OSA.

VOCAL CORD DYSFUNCTION

Vocal cord dysfunction (VCD) is characterized by paradoxical adduction of the vocal cords during inspiration that presents as breathlessness. Diagnosis of VCD is difficult since its clinical symptoms (dyspnea, wheeze) are common to those typically found in asthma. VCD may coexist with bronchial asthma or may be misdiagnosed as bronchial asthma. Diagnosis of VCD includes detailed history and physical examination, followed by spirometry and laryngoscopy.[13,14] It is characterized by truncation of the inspiratory limb of the flow-volume loop, though not a specific finding. In a study of 95 patients diagnosed with VCD, only 25% of the patients had this finding at baseline.[13] The standard criteria to diagnose VCD is direct observation of anterior vocal cord adduction during inspiratory phase, or during both inspiratory and expiratory phase, accompanied by a residual posterior glottic chink, using laryngoscopy (Fig. 9.3). These laryngoscopic findings along with respiratory symptoms confirm the diagnosis of VCD. However, being an invasive technique, it may

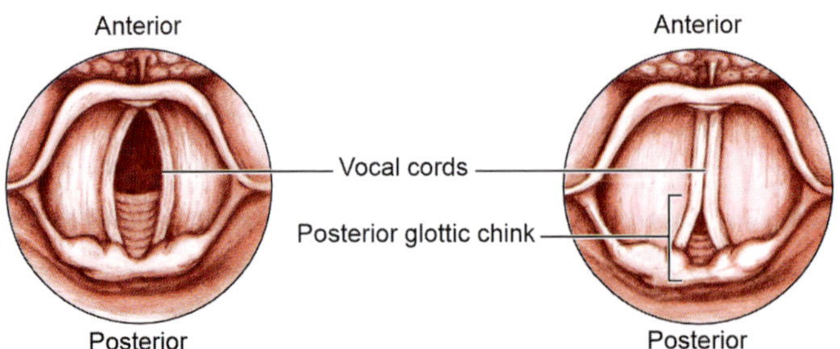

Fig. 9.3: Graphical representation of normal vocal cord abduction during inspiration (left) and paradoxical vocal cord adduction with a characteristic posterior "chink" in VCD (right)

cause upper airway irritation. A method of non-invasive assessment of glottic closure during the respiratory cycle in VCD could be of advantage.

Oscillometry methods have been studied as a non-invasive technique for the diagnosis of VCD. Oscillometry curve shows a signature spike in lung impedance with inspiration as detected by Z_5 (Fig. 9.4). Z_5 is the pulmonary impedance that includes both resistance and reactance at 5 Hz. D Komarow et al illustrated the difference in impedance tracing between VCD and voluntary glottic closure.[15]

OSCILLOMETRY IN CENTRAL AIRWAY OBSTRUCTION

Central airways refer to trachea and mainstem bronchi. Central airway obstruction (CAO) can occur due to a multitude of causes ranging from endoluminal obstruction by benign airway tumors, granulation tissue as in post-intubation tracheal stenosis (PITS), COVID associated tracheal stenosis (COATS), foreign body, airway stents, granulomatosis with polyangiitis; webs as in sub-glottic stenosis, tuberculosis; hyperdynamic airways as in tracheobronchomalacia, relapsing polychondritis; extrinsic compression by lymphadenopathy, vascular rings or aneurysm to endoluminal occlusion or extraluminal compression by malignant or metastatic tumors.

Spirometry studies are widely used to assess lung function in central airway obstruction. However, performing spirometry may not always be practical in patients with CAO due to patient related factors that interfere with an optimal forced expiratory maneuver (e.g. severe shortness of breath, excessive cough, fatigue, cognitive impairment, language differences, and lack of cooperation). Also, significant changes in spirometry values occur relatively late during airway obstruction and these values may not correlate with the degree of airway narrowing.

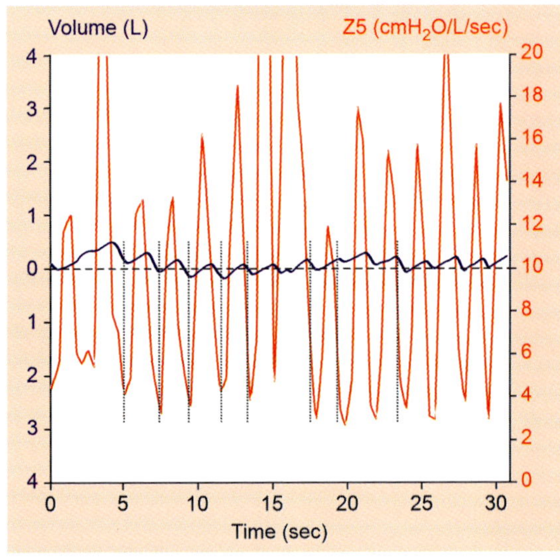

Fig. 9.4: Z_5 curve shows dramatic spike (>10 cm H$_2$O/L/sec) in impedance with onset of inspiration (vertical lines) correlated with vocal cord closure

Role of Oscillometry in Central Airway Osbtruction

1. **Non-invasive assessment of airway function:** Oscillometry is a non-invasive method that requires minimal patient effort and provides an estimation of the airway resistance and reactance at different frequencies.

2. **Identify the site and severity of obstruction:** It can identify the site of central airway obstruction and provide quantitative data on the airway resistance at different frequencies, thereby throwing light on the severity of obstruction as well.

3. **Monitor progression of airway obstruction:** A follow-up of oscillometry data can help monitor progression of the airway obstruction than doing repeated bronchoscopies or computed tomographs.

4. **Monitor treatment response:** It can be used to assess the effectiveness of intervention and treatment modalities used for central airway obstruction. It can also be used in planning treatment.

5. **Early detection of airway abnormalities in the central airways:** It can detect abnormalities in the central airways early on, before symptoms appear.

Oscillometry Parameters in Central Airway Obstruction

Oscillometry parameters in central airway obstruction are as follows:

1. Resistance at 5 Hz, R_5 increases
2. Resistance at 20 Hz, R_{20} increases (R_5 and R_{20} are on the same level)
3. R_{5-20} remains normal
4. Reactance at 5 Hz, X_5 remains normal
5. Area under the curve, A_x remains normal (*refer* to Fig. 9.1C).

Oscillometry techniques are a potential option in patients with suspected or known CAO who are unable to perform spirometry. It can help with treatment decision making, monitor progression, treatment response, proper documentation, and meaningful research. To understand the response of oscillometry at various levels and various degrees of obstruction, Xiuhua Si et al in 2021 evaluated the performance of an IOS system in 3D printed lung models with structural abnormalities at various locations with varying severities.[16] In a lung model with an airway extending up to the 6th generation, they studied IOS responses to three phenotypes of airway obstruction—varying glottic apertures, cardinal ridge tumours and segmental bronchial constrictions. R_{20} increased with the increase in the degree of airway obstructions. The slope of the R_{20} rise was higher with increasing cardinal ridge constrictions than bronchial constrictions. The resonant frequency dropped with the increase in the degree of obstruction for all three phenotypes. The variations of R_5 and X_5 were inconclusive in this study as these 3D-printed rigid casts cannot test airway compliance properties.

Yasuo et al studied the utility of the forced oscillation technique in evaluating the therapeutic result of tracheobronchial CAO in 12 patients, out of which 6 had a tracheal obstruction and 6 had a bronchial obstruction.[17] All oscillometry measurements R_5, R_{20}, R_{5-20}, F_{res}, X_5 and ALX (area under the curve) improved significantly post-interventional procedure. However, only the change in R_{20} significantly correlated with the change in minimum cross-sectional area (as measured by computed tomography image calculator) after intervention ($r = 0.6$, $p < 0.05$). An inverse correlation between tracheal narrowing and $X_5\%$ was also observed.[18]

A study on the assessment of CAO using impulse oscillometry before and after interventional bronchoscopy showed characteristic IOS curves differentiating fixed and variable central airway obstruction.[19] The variability of CAO was measured by collapsibility index, the percentage difference in airway lumen diameter between inspiration and expiration during quiet breathing calculated using morphometric bronchoscopy images. Fixed CAO was defined as a collapsibility index of <50% and variable CAO, as a collapsibility index of >50%. In fixed CAO, the airway resistance at 20 Hz showed a similar increase as resistance at 5 Hz, with respiratory reactance within normal range (Fig. 9.5A). In variable CAO (in the case of tracheobronchomalacia), the IOS curve showed frequency dependence of resistance and a decrease in respiratory reactance (Fig. 9.5B). The findings of variable CAO are like that of severe COPD; hence it is unclear whether IOS can differentiate between COPD patients with or without tracheobronchomalacia. Further studies are required to shed light on the role of oscillometry to distinguish between fixed and variable CAO, COPD patients with or without tracheobronchomalacia.

Dynamic airway collapse (DAC) of the larger airways is commonly seen during bronchoscopy. Oscillometric findings in DAC have been studied where patients who had DAC during bronchoscopy were made to perform IOS and spirometry. Patients with DAC had higher resonance frequency and greater fall in X_5, than those without DAC.[20]

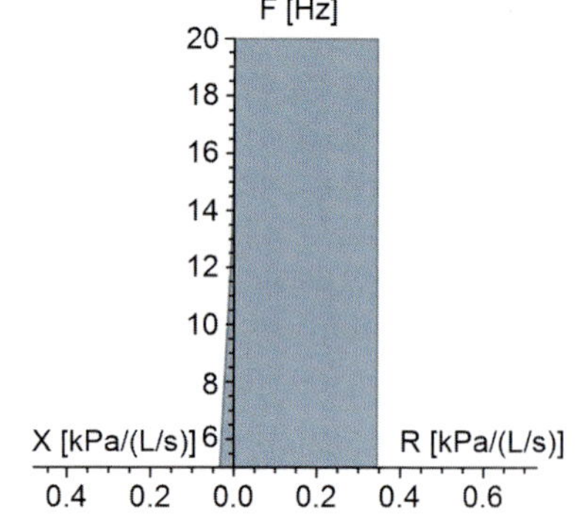

Fig. 9.5A: IOS curve in fixed CAO. Both R_5 and R_{20} are on the same level

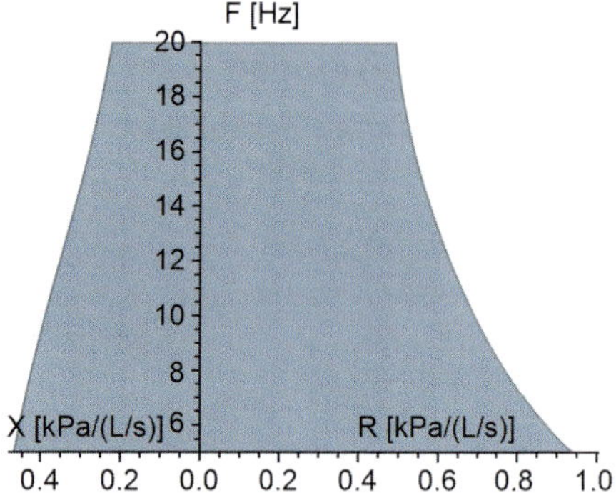

Fig. 9.5B: IOS curve in case of variable CAO shows frequency dependence of resistance and decrease in respiratory reactance

FUTURE DIRECTIONS

In the realm of respiratory medicine, the role of oscillometry in assessing and managing airway obstruction is poised for significant advancements. As we look ahead, several key directions are likely to expand the future and utility of this diagnostic technique. Further studies are required in describing the role of oscillometry in other causes of upper airway obstruction including chronic rhinosinusitis, laryngeal stenosis or foreign body aspiration, different types of sleep disordered breathing and more correlating oscillometry data with data from polysomnography. Further research is required to understand the role of oscillometry to distinguish between fixed and variable CAO, COPD patients with or without tracheobronchomalacia, and excessive dynamic airway collapse. The integration of artificial intelligence (AI) driven algorithms can help identify patterns and trends in airway obstruction that might be challenging for human interpretation without AI tools. This can help with personalized treatment plans and improved patient outcomes. To conclude, the future of oscillometry in the field of airway obstruction is marked by innovation, AI integration, improved accuracy, telemedicine applications, and interdisciplinary collaboration.

REFERENCES

1. Remmers JE, deGroot WJ, Sauerland EK, and Anch AM. Pathogenesis of Upper Airway Occlusion during Sleep. J Appl Physiol, 1978,44:931–38.

2. Shiota S, Ryan CM, Chiu KL, Ruttanaumpawan P, Haight J, Arzt M, Floras JS, Chan C, Bradley TD. Alterations in upper airway cross-sectional area in response to lower body positive pressure in healthy subjects. Thorax. 2007 Oct;62(10):868–72.

3. Montserrat JM, Farré R, Navajas D. New technologies to detect static and dynamic upper airway obstruction during sleep. Sleep Breath. 2001 Dec;5(4):193–206.

4. Farré R, Peslin R, Rotger M, Navajas D. Inspiratory dynamic obstruction detected by forced oscillation during CPAP. A model study. Am J Respir Crit Care Med. 1997 Mar;155(3):952–56.

5. Lorino AM, Lofaso F, Duizabo D, Zerah F, Goldenberg F, d'Ortho MP, Harf A, Lorino H. Respiratory resistive impedance as an index of airway obstruction during nasal continuous positive airway pressure titration. Am J Respir Crit Care Med. 1998 Nov;158(5 Pt 1):1465–70.

6. Navajas D, Farré R, Rotger M, Badia R, Puig-de-Morales M, Montserrat JM. Assessment of airflow obstruction during CPAP by means of forced oscillation in patients with sleep apnea. Am J Respir Crit Care Med. 1998 May;157(5 Pt 1):1526–30.

7. Albuquerque CGD, Andrade FMDD, Rocha MADA, Oliveira AFFD, Ladosky W, Victor EG, et al. Determining respiratory system resistance and reactance by impulse oscillometry in obese individuals. J Bras Pneumol. 2015 Oct;41(5):422–6.

8. Abdeyrim A, Tang L, Muhamat A, Abudeyrim K, Zhang Y, Li N, et al. Receiver operating characteristics of impulse oscillometry parameters for predicting obstructive sleep apnea in preobese and obese snorers. BMC Pulm Med. 2016 Aug 22;16(1):125.

9. Al-Alwan A, Bates JH, Chapman DG, et al. The nonallergic asthma of obesity. A matter of distal lung compliance. Am J Respir Crit Care Med 2014;189:1494–1502.

10. Cao X, Bradley TD, Bhatawadekar SA, et al. Effect of simulated obstructive apnea on thoracic fluid volume and airway narrowing in asthma. Am J Respir Crit Care Med 2021;203:908–10.

11. Salome CM, King GG, Berend N. Physiology of obesity and effects on lung function. J Appl Physiol 2010;108:206–11.

12. Jobin V, Rigau J, Beauregard J, Farre R, Monserrat J, Bradley TD, et al. Evaluation of upper airway patency during Cheyne–Stokes breathing in heart failure patients. Eur Respir J. 2012;40(6):1523–30.

13. Newman KB, Mason UG 3rd, Schmaling KB. Clinical features of vocal cord dysfunction. Am J Respir Crit Care Med. 1995;152:1382–6.

14. Morris MJ, Christopher KL. Diagnostic criteria for the classification of vocal cord dysfunction. Chest. 2010 Nov;138(5):1213–23.

15. Komarow HD, Young M, Nelson C, Metcalfe DD. Vocal cord dysfunction as demonstrated by impulse oscillometry. J Allergy Clin Immunol Pract. 2013 Jul-Aug;1(4):387–93.

16. Si X, Xi JS, Talaat M, Donepudi R, Su W-C, Xi J. Evaluation of Impulse Oscillometry in Respiratory Airway Casts with Varying Obstruction Phenotypes, Locations, and Complexities. Journal of Respiration. 2022; 2(1):44–58.

17. Yasuo M, Kitaguchi Y, Kinota F, Kosaka M, Urushihata K, Ushiki A, Yamamoto H, Kawakami S, Hanaoka M. Usefulness of the forced oscillation technique in assessing the therapeutic result of tracheobronchial central airway obstruction. Respir Investig. 2018 May;56(3):222–29.

18. Linhas R, Lima F, Coutinho D, Almeida J, Neves S, Oliveira A, et al. Role of the impulse oscillometry in the evaluation of tracheal stenosis. Pulmonology. 2018 Jul 1;24(4):224–30.

19. Handa H, Huang J, Murgu SD, Mineshita M, Kurimoto N, Colt HG, Miyazawa T. Assessment of central airway obstruction using impulse oscillometry before and after interventional bronchoscopy. Respir Care. 2014 Feb;59(2):231–40.

20. Impulse Oscillometry in Dynamic Airway Collapse—Novel Physiological Data. C41. New findings in pulmonary function. Am Thorac Soc Int Conf Meet Abstr Am Thorac Soc Int Conf Meet Abstr [Internet].

Oscillometry in Pediatrics

• *EV Krishnakumar*

Impulse oscillometry (IOS) is based on principles put forward by Dubois et al in 1956.[1] But still now IOS has not evolved as a robust tool in clinical medicine unlike spirometry. IOS continues to remain as a research tool even today. IOS has definite implications in many clinical conditions especially in the pediatric population. This chapter throws light into the implications of IOS in pediatric practice.

It is almost impossible to generate acceptable spirometry maneuvers from children less than six years of age.[2] IOS is a non-invasive technique that assesses the airways mechanically, using pressure fluctuations during tidal breathing. It can be used as an alternative tool to evaluate the lung function of children who cannot perform spirometry accurately.[3] Oscillations of small pressures are applied in the mouth and transmitted to the lungs. The resistance and reactance of respiratory system are thus calculated.[4] IOS can be applied in patients of all age groups. It is particularly beneficial in children since it is non-invasive, requires only tidal breathing and does not involve forced expiratory maneuvers.[5]

ASTHMA

IOS is very useful in assessing children with asthma.[6] In asthmatic patients there is an increase in airway resistance, especially in the peripheral airways.[7] In IOS tracings, asthmatic patients show increased R_5 values, compared with controls, especially during exacerbation.[8] Other findings include normal R_{20}, more negative X_5, and increase in F_{res}.[9] Among the various IOS parameters, the most sensitive ones to detect airway obstruction and to evaluate the severity of asthma and its exacerbations are R_5, R_{5-20} and A_x.[10] R_{5-20} and A_x may be useful for early detection of pulmonary function abnormalities.[11]

IOS AND SPIROMETRY

Many studies have evaluated the corelation between the results of IOS and spirometry in children. In these studies, there is a significant correlation between IOS parameters and spirometric indices especially FEV_1.[12] Compared with spirometric indices, IOS parameters are more sensitive in identifying patients with asthma and excluding those without asthma.[13] IOS is also useful in following up these asthmatic patients. It may detect airway obstruction earlier than spirometry.[14]

BRONCHODILATOR RESPONSE

Many studies have shown that IOS is better than spirometry when assessing the bronchodilator response, an important predictor of who will respond to pharmacotherapy and who will not. R_5 is the main parameter to evaluate the bronchodilator response.[15] The best cut-off for positive bronchodilator response in IOS is unclear. Various studies show a decrease in R_5 values ranging from 20 to 50%.[16]

ASTHMA CONTROL

IOS can be used to assess the level of control of asthma. Studies reveal that R_{5-20} and A_x can correctly classify asthma control in more than 80% of the studied population. We can suspect the loss of asthma control in patients with increased R_{5-20} and A_x—which are parameters that assess the peripheral airways.[17] Decreased airway calibre and increased airway muscle tone contribute to the onset of symptoms in asthmatic children.

BRONCHIAL PROVOCATION TESTING

There is evidence that an increase of 50% of baseline R_5 values show a significant correlation with a 20% fall in FEV_1. This can be made use of in bronchial provocation testing.[18] Increase in resistance values precede the fall in FEV_1. This makes IOS a tool with better sensitivity than spirometry in detecting bronchoconstriction induced by methacholine or allergens.[19]

RESPONSE TO TREATMENT OF ASTHMA

The IOS parameter that can be used to assess the response to asthma treatment is reactance area (A_x). Studies show that there is a steady and continuous improvement of A_x during the long-term follow-up of asthmatic children who are on optimal treatment. After initiation of treatment, improvement in lung function can be identified early by IOS.[20]

PRETERM BIRTH AND BRONCHOPULMONARY DYSPLASIA

Oscillometry is a clinically useful measure of lung function in children who have survived from very preterm birth. In comparison with preschoolers delivered at term, the preterm ones have increased R_{rs}, more negative X_{rs} and increased area of reactance (A_x) and resonant frequency (F_{res}). In preterm babies with bronchopulmonary dysplasia (BPD), the deficits are even greater. In very preterm infants on noninvasive respiratory support, X_{rs} measured in the first week of life has been shown to improve prognostication of respiratory outcome. Abnormalities in oscillometric parameters persist up to at least adolescence.[21]

IOS IN CYSTIC FIBROSIS

In patients with cystic fibrosis, R_5, R_{20}, F_{res}, and AX values increase, and X_5 values decrease during the period of exacerbation. After successful treatment of exacerbation, these values return to baseline.[22]

MISCELLANEOUS INDICATIONS

Researchers have used IOS to detect decreased lung function due to early infection by rhinovirus (before three years of age). X_5 was reduced, which was confirmed by spirometry values.[23]

When patients with post-infectious bronchiolitis obliterans were assessed with IOS, the values of Z_5, R_5 increased and X_5 was more negative. These indicate an increase in the peripheral airway resistance.[24]

In children with congenital malformations, reactance values are increased when compared to controls.[25]

In the respiratory evaluation of adenosine deaminase deficiency—severe combined immunodeficiency (ADA-SCID), IOS has a role. Patients demonstrate alterations in the peripheral airways. This is indicated by the measurement of resistance and reactance at low frequencies (R_5, R_{10}, and X_5).[26]

In 50% of patients with GERD oesophagitis, IOS demonstrates increased airway resistance (R_5 and R_{20}) despite having normal spirometry.[27]

In obese children, despite having normal spirometry indices, IOS may show evidence of abnormal lung function, probably since it assesses distal airways in a better manner.[28]

In critically ill children, oscillometry may be useful for monitoring the effects of positional changes and adjustment of PEEP. In extremely preterm newborns receiving invasive ventilation, IOS is useful to improve prediction of respiratory outcomes.[29]

LIMITATIONS

While performing IOS, patients should avoid chewing movements, vocalization, and swallowing, as well as placing the tongue inside the mouthpiece. Very young children (less than 3 years old) and those who have attention deficit may not be able to perform this test properly. Moreover, clinicians may find it difficult to interpret the results of IOS, since it is not routinely used in clinical practice. Lack of inadequate range of normal values and the high cost of IOS equipment are other limitations in using IOS.

REFERENCES

1. Dubois A, Brody A, Lewis D, Burgess B Jr. Oscillation mechanics of lungs and chest in man. J Appl Physiol. 1956;8:587–94.
2. Guilbert T, Singh A, Danov Z, Evans M, Jackson D, Burton R, et al. Decreased lung function after preschool wheezing rhinovirus illnesses in children at risk to develop asthma. J Allergy Clin Immunol. 2011;128:532–8.
3. Escobar H, Carver TW Jr. Pulmonary function testing in young children. Curr Allergy Asthma Rep. 2011;11:473–81.
4. Goldman MD. Clinical application of forced oscillation. Pulm Pharmacol Ther. 2001;14:341–50.
5. Al-Mutairi S, Sharma P, Al-Alawi A, Al-Deen J. Impulse oscillometry: an alternative modality to the conventional pulmonary function test to categorize obstructive pulmonary disorders. Clin Exp Med. 2007;7:56–64.
6. Knihtila H, Kotaniemi-Syrjanen A, Makela M, Bondestam J, Pelkonen A, Malmberg L. Preschool oscillometry and lung function at adolescence in asthmatic children. Pediatr Pulmonol. 2015;50:1205–13.
7. Kaczka D, Dellacá R. Oscillation mechanics of the respiratory system: applications to lung disease. Crit Rev Biomed Eng. 2011;39:337–59.
8. Batmaz S, Kuyucu S, Arıkoglu T, Tezol O, Aydogdu A. Impulse oscillometry in acute and stable asthmatic children: a comparison with spirometry. J Asthma. 2015;14:1–8.
9. Gochicoa-Rangel L, Cantú-González G, Miguel-Reyes J, Rodríguez-Moreno L, Torre-Bouscoulet L. Oscilometría deimpulso: recomendaciones y procedimiento. Neumol Cir Torax. 2014;73:138–49.
10. Batmaz S, Kuyucu S, Arıkoglu T, Tezol O, Aydogdu A. Impulse oscillometry in acute and stable asthmatic children: a comparison with spirometry. J Asthma. 2015;14:1–8.
11. Meraz E, Nazeran H, Ramos C, Nava P, Diong B, Goldman M. Analysis of impulse oscillometric measures of lung function and respiratory system model parameters in small airway-impaired and healthy children over a 2-year period. BioMed Eng OnLine. 2011;10:21.

12. Batmaz S, Kuyucu S, Arıkoglu T, Tezol O, Aydogdu A. Impulse oscillometry in acute and stable asthmatic children: a comparison with spirometry. J Asthma. 2015;14:1–8.

13. Komarow H, Skinner J, Young M, Gaskins D, Nelson C, Gergen P, et al. A study of the use of impulse oscillometry in the evaluation of children with asthma: analysis of lung parameters, order effect, and utility compared with spirometry. Pediatr Pulmonol. 2012;47:18–26.

14. Galant SP, Komarow HD, Shin HW, Siddiqui S, Lipworth BJ. The case for impulse oscillometry in the management of asthma in children and adults. Ann Allergy Asthma Immunol. 2017;118:664–71.

15. Diong B, Singh K, Menendez R. Effects of two inhaled corticosteroid/long-acting beta-agonist combinations on small airway dysfunction in mild asthmatics measured by impulse oscillometry. J Asthma Allergy. 2013;6:109–16.

16. Klug B, Bisgaard H. Specific airway resistance, interrupter resistance, and respiratory impedance in healthy children aged 2–7 years. Pediatric Pulmonol. 1998;25:322–31.

17. PP de Oliveira Jorgea, b, JHP de Limab, DC Chong e Silva c, d, D Medeirose, D Soléb, GF Wandalsenb. Impulse oscillometry in the assessment of children's lung function. Allergol Immunopathol (Madr). 2019;47(3):295–302.

18. Naji N, Keung E, Kane J, Watson RM, Killian KJ, Gauvreau GM. Comparison of changes in lung function measured by plethysmography and IOS after bronchoprovocation. Respir Med. 2013;107:503–10.

19. Schulze J, Smith HJ, Fuchs J, Herrmann E, Dressler M, Rose MA, et al. Methacholine challenge in young children as evaluated by spirometry and impulse oscillometry. Respir Med. 2012;106:627–34.

20. Larsen GL, Morgan W, Heldt GP, Mauger DT, Boehmer SJ, Chinchilli VM, et al. Impulse oscillometry versus spirometry in a long-term study of controller therapy for pediatric asthma. J Allergy Clin Immunol. 2009;123:861–7.

21. Kaminsky DA, Simpson SJ, Berger KI, et al. Clinical significance and applications of oscillometry. Eur Respir Rev 2022;31:210208 [DOI: 10.1183/16000617.0208-2021].

22. Sakarya A, Uyan ZS, Baydemir C, Anık Y, Erdem E, Gokdemir Y, et al. Evaluation of children with cystic fibrosis by impulse oscillometry when stable and at exacerbation. Pediatr Pulmonol. 2016;51:1151–8.

23. Guilbert T, Singh A, Danov Z, Evans M, Jackson D, Burton R, et al. Decreased lung function after preschool wheezing rhinovirus illnesses in children at risk to develop asthma. J Allergy Clin Immunol. 2011;128:532–8.

24. Li Y, Liu L, Qiao H, Cheng H, Cheng H. Post-infectious bronchiolitis obliterans in children: a review of 42 cases. BMC Pediatr. 2014;14:238.

25. Mandaliya P, Morten M, Kumar R, James A, Deshpande A, Murphy V, et al. Ventilation inhomogeneities in children with congenital thoracic malformations. BMC Pulm Med. 2015;15:25.

26. Komarow H, Sokolic R, Hershfield M, Kohn D, Young M, Metcalfe D, et al. Impulse oscillometry identifies peripheral airway dysfunction in children with adenosine deaminase deficiency. Orphanet J Rare Dis. 2015;10:159.

27. Eidani E, Hashemi S, Raji H, Askarabadi M. A Comparison of impulse oscillometry and spirometry values in patients with gastroesophageal reflux disease. Middle East J Dig Dis. 2013;5:22–8.

28. Assumpc̦ão MS, Ribeiro JD, Wamosy RM, Figueiredo FC, Parazzi PL, Schivinski CI. Impulse oscillometry and obesity in children. J Pediatr (Rio J). 2017.

29. Veneroni C, Wallström L, Sindelar R, et al. Oscillatory respiratory mechanics on the first day of life improves prediction of respiratory outcomes in extremely preterm newborns. Pediatr Res 2019;85:312–17.

A Practical Approach of Impulse Oscillometry

• *Akhil Paul*

Spirometry serves as a major tool for a clinician in diagnosing and following up various obstructive and restrictive lung disorders. But, as spirometry measures forced inspiratory and expiratory volumes, the quality of the values and thus the test depends a lot on the patient and his or her efforts. In a research study done by Van De Hei et al on the clinical use of spirometry, the quality and the diagnostic value, the general practitioners and the pulmonologists stated that spirometry was clinically useful in more than eighty-eight per cent of the cases.[1] But agreement on the diagnosis was very low and only thirteen per cent of the spirometry tests had fulfilled the ATS/ERS criteria. Impulse oscillometry becomes a better choice in this aspect as it requires only tidal breaths from the patient.

ADVANTAGES OF IMPULSE OSCILLOMETRY

1. Only tidal breath is required (no forced maneuvers)
2. Only a minimal patient co-operation is required
3. Can be performed even in children not <2 years of age[2]
4. Can be performed in patients with neuromuscular diseases, intellectual disabilities, post-cardiothoracic surgery, etc.[3]
5. High sensitivity in detecting peripheral airway obstruction.

CLINICAL APPLICATION OF IMPULSE OSCILLOMETRY

- Because of the very high sensitivity of the impulse oscillometry in detecting the distal airway obstruction, this technique is very handy in making a diagnosis, where the clinical suspicion is questioned by a normal spirometry.[4]
- Bronchodilator reversibility using inhaled short acting β_2-agonists or short acting muscarinic antagonists can be assessed.
- It is feasible to perform oscillometry in elderly, children, patients with neuromuscular disorders[5], impaired intellect, mechanically ventilated patients[6] and even during sleep[2].
- Aerosol generation during various procedures was a major concern during the COVID-19 pandemic. It is risk that need to be handled carefully during any viral pandemic like COVID-19 or influenza. Healthcare facilities had stopped performing spirometry during the pandemic period because of this particular reason. But oscillometry being an unforced procedure, aerosol generation during the same is very low and hence it can be performed without any significant added risk.[7]

- Oscillometry has proven to be having a great potential in diagnosing and monitoring various respiratory diseases other than the obstructive airway diseases like cystic fibrosis,[8] interstitial lung diseases,[9] bronchopulmonary dysplasia,[10] bronchiolitis obliterans in lung transplant recipients,[11] vocal cord dysfunction,[12] etc.

The variability on repetition of all impulse oscillometry parameters significantly higher (~10%) compared to FEV_1 (~5%). But they are clinically acceptable. At the same time the impulse oscillometry parameters are more repeatable than other common spirometry parameters like FEF50 (~20%).[13]

A CLINICAL ALGORITHM

Step 1

> **Indication:**
> - Spirometry is indicated, but the patient is unable to perform spirometry.
> - Spirometry results are not able to contribute to a diagnosis which can explain the respiratory symptoms of the patient.

Step 2

> **Prerequisite:**
> - Off short acting β_2-agonist (SABA) for 4 hours
> - Off long acting β_2-agonist (LABA) for 24 hours

Step 3

> **Calibration:**
> - As per the instructions of the manufacturer

Step 4

> **Patient positioning:**
> - Sitting position
> - Legs uncrossed to decrease the extrathoracic pressures
> - Nose clip
> - Mouthpiece at an optimum height
> - Neck comfortably extended
> - Leak prevented by a tight seal between the lips and the mouthpiece
> - Cheeks firmly held as impedance of cheek, tongue and upper airway will affect R_{19-20}

Step 5

> **Procedure:**
> - Impulse oscillometry is performed
> - Minimum 3 acceptable readings (pre- and post-bronchodilator) taken
> - Age and height matched control used

Step 6

> **Validity:**
> - Variation in consecutive R_5 values should be less than 15%

Step 7

<table>
<tr><td colspan="4">Interpretation using parameters:
A. Obstructive disease</td></tr>
<tr><td>R_5</td><td>R_{19-20}</td><td>R_{5-20}</td><td>Interpretation</td></tr>
<tr><td>Increased</td><td>Increased</td><td>Normal</td><td>Central airway obstruction</td></tr>
<tr><td>Increased</td><td>Normal</td><td>Increased</td><td>Peripheral airway obstruction</td></tr>
<tr><td>Highly increased</td><td>Increased</td><td>Increased</td><td>Total airway obstruction</td></tr>
</table>

<table>
<tr><td colspan="2">Reversibility criteria:</td></tr>
<tr><td>Parameter</td><td>Change after bronchodilator</td></tr>
<tr><td>R_5</td><td>40%</td></tr>
<tr><td>X_5</td><td>50%</td></tr>
<tr><td>A_x</td><td>80%</td></tr>
<tr><td>F_{res}</td><td>Leftward shift</td></tr>
</table>

B. Restrictive disease:
- More negative X_5 and increased F_{res} with normal R

Interpretation using graphics:
- Increased R_5, more negative X_5 and increased F_{res}: Peripheral airway obstruction
- Increased R_5 and R_{19-20} with normal X_5 and F_{res}: Central airway obstruction
- Normal R_5, More negative X_5 and increased F_{res}: Restrictive lung disease

Limitations

- Even though impulse oscillometry is based on breaths at tidal volume, a minimum co-operation from the patient is still required.
- If the cheeks are not supported well, it can falsely decrease the resistance values.[14]
- Standardization of different types of machine need to be done.
- Reference values for different population need to be established and validated.
- Reference cut-off for significant reversibility using bronchodilator needs to be validated using larger studies.
- Larger clinical trials are required to establish and standardize the role of impulse oscillometry in restrictive lung disease, vocal cord dysfunction and in ventilated or sedated patients.
- Portability and the cost of the device is a limitation in resource limited settings. But more compact and cheaper versions of oscillometry devices are now at various stages of development and marketing.

Spirometry is better studied and more widely accepted at present.[15] So, the interpretation is comparatively easier for the practitioner. Clinical application of IOS parameters are still studied in various pulmonary diseases. The reference values for IOS in various populations are yet to be standardized and the results of the ongoing trials will contribute to that.[16] During bronchoprovocation testing, the changes in R_{rs} and A_x were detected much before any change in FEV_1 was noticed.[17] In obese asthmatics, greater expiratory flow limitation associated with bronchial challenge can be measured better by X_{rs} than FEV_1.[18]

As we are at a transition phase regarding the pulmonary function tests, it is wiser to perform spirometry as well as the impulse oscillometry in each patient. Apart from the fact that both tests can act complimentarily, performing both the tests and analysing the parameters will give a better knowledge regarding the underlying lung disease and will provide more informative data for comparative studies in the future. While performing tests requiring deep breaths (e.g. FeNO, spirometry, DLCO) along with oscillometry, later should be performed at first prior to other tests, as deep breathing can worsen the obstruction measured by the oscillometry as well as the spirometry.[19,20]

REFERENCES

1. van de Hei, SJ, Flokstra-de Blok, BMJ, Baretta, HJ et al. Quality of spirometry and related diagnosis in primary care with a focus on clinical use. npj Prim. Care Respir. Med. 30, 22 (2020). https://doi.org/10.1038/s41533-020-0177-z

2. Beydon N, Davis SD, Lombardi E, Allen JL, Arets HG, Aurora P, et al. An official American Thoracic Society/ European Respiratory Society statement: Pulmonary function testing in preschool children. Am J Respir Crit Care Med. 2007;175:1304–45.

3. Desiraju K, Agrawal A. Impulse oscillometry: The state-of-art for lung function testing. Lung India. 2016;33:410–6.

4. Oppenheimer BW, Goldring RM, Herberg ME, Hofer IS, Reyfman PA, Liautaud S, et al. Distal airway function in symptomatic subjects with normal spirometry following world trade center dust exposure. Chest. 2007;132:1275–82.

5. Morgan WJ, Stern DA, Sherrill DL, Guerra S, Holberg CJ, Guilbert TW, et al. Outcome of asthma and wheezing in the first 6 years of life: Follow-up through adolescence. Am J Respir Crit Care Med. 2005;172:1253–8.

6. Handa H, Huang J, Murgu SD, Mineshita M, Kurimoto N, Colt HG, Miyazawa T. Assessment of central airway obstruction using impulse oscillometry before and after interventional bronchoscopy. Respir Care 2014;59(2):231–40.

7. Torregiani C, Veneroni C, Confalonieri P, Citton GM, Salton F, Jaber M, et al. (2022) Monitoring respiratory mechanics by oscillometry in COVID-19 patients receiving non-invasive respiratory support. PLoS ONE 17(3): e0265202. https://doi.org/10.1371/journal.pone.0265202

8. Shok-Yin Lee, Judith Morton, Sally Chapman, Emily Hopkins, Chien-Li Holmes-Liew, Lauren Bussell, Is impulse oscillometry (IOS) better than spirometry for monitoring treatment outcomes in adult cystic fibrosis (CF) pulmonary exacerbations? A pilot study. European Respiratory Journal 2019 54: PA335; DOI: 10.1183/13993003.congress-2019.PA335

9. Cheng WC, Chang SH, Chen WC, Wu BR, Chen CH, Lin CC, Hsu WH, Lan JL, Chen DY. Application of impulse oscillometry to detect interstitial lung disease and airway disease in adults with rheumatoid arthritis. BMC Pulm Med. 2023 Sep 8;23(1):331. doi: 10.1186/s12890-023-02615-0. PMID: 37684581; PMCID: PMC10485984.

10. Shannon Gunawardana, Christopher Harris, Anne Greenough, Use of impulse oscillometry to assess lung function in prematurely born children and young people: Comparisons with spirometry, Paediatric Respiratory Reviews, Volume 45, 2023, Pages 52-57, ISSN 1526-0542, https://doi.org/10.1016/j.prrv.2022.07.003.

11. Crowhurst, Thomas D. MBBS1,2; Butler, Jessica A. MBBS1; Bussell, Lauren A. MMSc1; Johnston, Sonya D. PhD1; Yeung, David PhD2,3; Hodge, Greg PhD1,2; Snell, Greg I. MD4,5; Yeo, Aeneas MBBS1,2; Holmes, Mark MD2,6; Holmes-Liew, Chien-Li MCSc2,6. Impulse Oscillometry Versus Spirometry to Detect Bronchiolitis Obliterans Syndrome in Bilateral Lung Transplant Recipients: A Prospective Diagnostic Study. Transplantation ():10.1097/TP.0000000000004868, December 04, 2023. | DOI: 10.1097/TP.0000000000004868

12. Jordi Rigau, Ramon Farré, Xavier Trepat, Dennis Shusterman, Daniel Navajas, Oscillometric assessment of airway obstruction in a mechanical model of vocal cord dysfunction, Journal of Biomechanics, Volume 37, Issue 1, 2004, Pages 37–43, ISSN 0021-9290, https://doi.org/10.1016/S0021-9290(03)00256-2.

13. Koundinya Desiraju and Anurag Agrawal. Impulse oscillometry: The state-of-art for lung function testing. Lung India. 2016 Jul-Aug; 33(4): 410–416. doi: 10.4103/0970-2113.184875

14. Desiraju K, Agrawal A. Impulse oscillometry: The state-of-art for lung function testing. Lung India. 2016 Jul-Aug;33(4):410-6. doi: 10.4103/0970-2113.184875. PMID: 27578934; PMCID: PMC4948229.

15. Pellegrino R, Viegi G, Brusasco V, et al. Interpretative strategies for lung function tests. *Eur Respir J.* 2005; 26(5):948–968.

16. Lennart KA. Lundblad, Salman Siddiqui, Ynuk Bossé and Ronald J. Dandurand (2021) Applications of oscillometry in clinical research and practice, Canadian Journal of Respiratory, Critical Care, and Sleep Medicine, 5:1, 54 68, DOI: 10.1080/24745332.2019.1649607

17. Berger KI, Kalish S, Shao Y, et al. Isolated small airway reactivity during bronchoprovocation as a mechanism for respiratory symptoms in WTC dust-exposed community members. *Am J Ind Med* 2016; 59: 767–776. doi:10.1002/ajim.22639

18. Rory Chan, Brian Lipworth, Clinical impact of obesity on oscillometry lung mechanics in adults with asthma, Annals of Allergy, Asthma and Immunology, Volume 131, Issue 3, 2023, Pages 338-342.e3, ISSN 1081-1206, https://doi.org/10.1016/j.anai.2023.05.014.

19. Jensen A, Atileh H, Suki B, et al. Selected contribution: airway caliber in healthy and asthmatic subjects: effects of bronchial challenge and deep inspirations. *J Appl Physiol* 2001; 91: 506–515. doi:10.1152/jappl.2001.91.1.506

20. Slats AM, Janssen K, van Schadewijk A, et al. Bronchial inflammation and airway responses to deep inspiration in asthma and chronic obstructive pulmonary disease. *Am J Respir Crit Care Med* 2007; 176: 121–128. doi:10.1164/rccm.200612-1814OC

Future Prospects of Oscillometry

• *Lennart KA Lundblad* • *Charu Singh*

It is commonplace to explore extended use of any new technology, and oscillometry is, of course, not an exception. While looking into the crystal ball might be deceiving and even create false hopes, there are a few areas where respiratory oscillometry likely will be useful outside of the traditional and common respiratory diseases such as asthma, COPD, and ILD. In addition, we can also anticipate expanded use of the technology for disease monitoring outside of the traditional healthcare settings such as in the patient's own home. There are also several types of respiratory tests regularly performed to elucidate the condition of a patient's lung health using spirometry which might be possible to perform quicker, easier and with higher precision using oscillometry.

Oscillometry is being extensively used in animal models of human lung diseases and to test drug targets, hence it is likely that some of the utility in the laboratory will make its way into the clinic eventually.[1]

In this chapter, we will cover some use of oscillometry that is already established in some centers, but which deserve broader use. In the latter part of the chapter, we will discuss expanded uses of oscillometry where there are fewer publications but where we can see the potential in the future. Hopefully, this will be an inspiration for further development of the technology.

LUNG TRANSPLANT MONITORING

Acute cellular rejection (ACR) is common during the initial 3 months after lung transplant and is cause for serious concern and intervention with immunosuppressing drugs. As with any lung inflammation early detection is very important to allow for timely interventions to take place. Recent discoveries suggest that oscillometry could detect ACR much earlier than spirometry and before any symptoms are noticed. Out of 138 patients there were 16 episodes of ACR all of which were detected by oscillometry and only one with spirometry. The study also demonstrated a return to normal lung function post-treatment.[2] Assuming this is confirmed in future studies this holds promise for a change in the practice of monitoring this group of vulnerable patients.[3,4]

A common end-stage condition of transplanted lungs is known as chronic lung allograft dysfunction (CLAD), which carries a poor survival rate. Furthermore, patients who have poor baseline lung allograft dysfunction (BLAD) are at higher risk to have a poor survival rate. Recent findings suggest that respiratory oscillometry, in particular abnormal elastance, is an important physiologic feature to detect both BLAD and CLAD.[5–7]

Manifesting in ways that resembles transplant rejections bronchiolitis obliterans is commonly seen in patients who have received bone marrow cell transplants. The mechanism behind this is still not understood but the condition and treatment are similar to that of ACR in lung transplant cases. Monitoring this group of patients with oscillometry has the potential to further improve their care and increase survival.[8]

Thus, oscillometry can identify physiological changes associated with ACR and CLAD that are not otherwise detectable using spirometry and could be useful for graft monitoring after a lung transplant. While there are limited number of publications at this time, the data compelling rationale for incorporating oscillometry as an adjunct to spirometry for patient monitoring after lung transplant. Any findings with oscillometry will have to be confirmed with bronchoscopy and transbronchial biopsy and infections ruled out or treated before immunosuppressant therapy is initiated. It remains to be shown that early detection of ACR will improve survival, though the suspicion is that it will.[3]

CHALLENGE TESTING

Challenge testing can take on several shapes and are commonplace in diagnosing and monitoring patients with various respiratory pathologies. A challenge test can be used to aid in ruling in or ruling out certain conditions or establishing the efficacy of an intervention.

Reversibility

One of the most common tests used is the reversibility test in asthma. Typically done using spirometry it includes establishing the patients baseline lung function and then administering a dose of an inhaled bronchodilator, a β-agonist or a muscarinic antagonist, then do another lung function test. If the patient is reversible the lung function will have improved; the traditional cut-off used is an increase in FEV_1 of 12%.[9] This is also possible to do using oscillometry in an analogous way; a baseline measurement followed by administration of a bronchodilator and then a post-bronchodilator measurement, and then calculating the % change from baseline. Because several parameters are generated from an impedance measurement, the current technical recommendation from ERS suggests different cut-offs for different parameters.[10] There are, however, competing opinions about what constitutes a significant shift from baseline, thus the user is strongly encouraged to monitor the literature on this topic as the cut-offs are likely to change or might be different for different patient categories (e.g. children vs adults, or age).[11–13]

A novel drug, an interesting use of the reversibility test that was recently been proposed, is to test a patient's degree of reversibility while under regular treatment for asthma. The notion is that if a patient remains reversible despite being treated there is room for improvement. In a study by Cottee et al,[14] it was found that oscillometry was better than spirometry in detecting bad asthma control as defined by them having significant reversibility despite being under treatment. A bronchodilator response was identified more frequently with oscillometry than with spirometry in 54% vs 27% of the test subjects. They also found that the reactance parameter A_x (a measure of elastance) identified more patients with poor asthma control than did spirometry with 69% vs 41%. This report thus suggests a novel way of using a combination of a bronchodilator challenge with sensitive oscillometry to monitor asthmatic patients. In another study the same group studied asthma control in patients with or without fixed airway obstruction and showed that the reactance parameters had a stronger and more consistent association with asthma symptoms than did spirometry, this was independent of how severe the airflow limitation was.[15] The findings support the notion that oscillometry is a relevant test and could help with the assessment of asthma, and an abnormal bronchodilator response is sensitive in identifying poor asthma control. It should be noted that asthmatics likely have more of a bronchodilator response than do COPD patients.[16]

We like to posit that reversibility testing could also be a powerful test in clinical drug studies where it could help with optimizing the dose to use to treat and determining the overall efficacy of a drug candidate. If patients under treatment with a drug candidate are significantly reversible, then there would still be room for improvement, if they do not reverse any further, they are likely to be well controlled.

Hyperresponsiveness

Another common challenge test is to determine the patient's response to bronchoconstriction, most commonly elicited by letting the test subject inhale incremental doses of methacholine and then measuring the response after each dose and calculating the % change from the baseline. These tests are often referred to as testing for hyperresponsiveness or hyper-reactivity. This is relatively common test using spirometry but oscillometry is also well suited for this kind of assessment, as demonstrated in the early days of oscillometry.[17–19] As with the reversibility test discussed above, it is vitally important to establish a correct baseline. Once that baseline has been established the test subject would start the methacholine inhalation protocol and a measurement will be performed after each dose and the change in impedance parameters calculated. The traditional cut-off for spirometry is known as a PC20. Publications comparing spirometry and oscillometry suggest different values for the oscillometry parameters, maybe because children and adults do not have the same sensibility towards methacholine.[20–24] A consensus on the cut-off for oscillometry that corresponds to that of spirometry is needed and it might be different for different patient categories.

Importantly oscillometry has been used to elucidate hyperresponsiveness in children and found to be safe and useful.[25] This is important because children often have problems performing spirometry, hence this opens up the possibility to assess them and aid with diagnosing asthma.

Because oscillometry is agnostic as to what might have caused a change in lung function, it is reasonable to believe that other mediators than methacholine will elicit responses that can be registered by measuring respiratory impedance. The most common alternative today is the mannitol challenge. While mannitol is less common this does not matter for the measurement, if there is a bronchial reaction the oscillometer will register the change in lung mechanics.[21]

While methacholine challenge has been used with oscillometry it is not a widespread practise. With better software integration and increased awareness, we think that responsiveness testing using oscillometry will be an important tool for the clinician going forward.

SELF-MONITORING

Self-monitoring using hand-held spirometers is relatively common. If the patient is properly trained to perform the measurement this can be a great help in ascertaining that the disease is properly managed and might give an indication when the patient is deteriorating. The problem is that the outcome of the test is highly dependent on the effort by the patient. If oscillometry were to be developed to include individual use outside of the healthcare clinic some of those issues might be avoided just because oscillometry is much less dependent on the test subjects' interaction with the device. As described in the previous chapters the subject just needs to do tidal breathing into the device and supporting their cheeks while the device carries out the measurement. It should thus be possible to train most patients to do measurements on their own with a little to no risk of errors, in particular if the device has some sort of quality assessment built in.

The next issue to be addressed is the interpretation of the result. Should it be up to the patient to understand the result, or should the device have built-in interpretation algorithms, a third possibility is that the device communicates with the healthcare provider to have an interpretation done. Of course, one could conceivably have a combination of all possibilities. The goal would be to provide the user with feedback about their lung health condition such that they can make adequate adjustments with respect to interventions and hopefully avoid an exacerbation.

There are published studies exploring home use oscillometry devices to elucidate the risk of having an exacerbation of asthma though we are still waiting to see full commercialization of the technology. In a study by Wong et al,[26] they showed that teenagers with asthma were able to successfully perform measurements at home and just looking at very basic parameters (R_5 and X_5) they were able to indicate when an exacerbation was approaching. Interestingly, the study indicated that the participants were happy doing the oscillometry measurements but frequently skipped their medication.

Home oscillometry has also been used for early detection of exacerbations in COPD.[27] They found that changes in oscillometry might precede an exacerbation by as much as three days leading to the conclusion that oscillometry might be a sensitive biomarker for early detection of an exacerbation.

Perhaps the most powerful use of home-oscillometry would be to use the technology as a telemonitoring tool allowing the healthcare providers to intervene when signs of an imminent exacerbation are detected.[28]

Other Potential Uses for Oscillometry

In the preclinical settings it is common to use oscillometry to detect lesions caused by any number of interventions[1,29] and safety pharmacology is one area where oscillometry is used before moving a drug candidate to human testing. In many cases, drugs receive conditional approval and sometimes there is reason to expect side effects on the lungs. One example is fibrosis caused by cytostatic drugs such as bleomycin, but drug-induced interstitial complications are relatively common but might be difficult to detect.[30] It remains to be shown that oscillometry is sensitive and specific to such lesions but recent advances in detecting interstitial lesions of other origins show promise in this regard.[31]

Intensive care often involves intubation and respiratory support by a ventilator. While this is a life-saving intervention it also comes with great risk of inducing additional injury by ventilator-induced lung injury and safe ventilation strategies are essential to protect the lung from further injury.[32] Research is underway using oscillometry to assess safe ventilation strategies with the hope of decreasing time on ventilator and ultimately increasing ICU survival rates.[33]

CHILDREN AND INFANTS

The use of oscillometry in young children has long been recognized as a distinct advantage over spirometry, young children often have difficulty understanding or performing the necessary maneuvers to render quality spirometry results.[34] Because oscillometry only requires a minimum of cooperation by the test subject it is considered feasible to use in young children and numerous publications support its use.[35–40]

Compared with toddlers, testing lung function in infants comes with a number of obstacles where often the infant has had to be sedated, placed in a plethysmograph, and then forced maneuvers were induced by compressing the infant's chest to generate the equivalent of a spirometry measurement. It goes without saying that this is a highly specialized procedure and one that not many centers are capable of doing, hence the need to warrant better methods.

Recently oscillometry equipment has been developed allowing experimental studies in infants, and so far, results look promising, at least in terms of feasibility. It has been shown that oscillometry can safely be done in newborn and there is even data from prematurely born infants.[41–43] Measurements are typically done during regular sleep, which of course introduces the problem of not arousing the infant lest the measurement might be compromised. The posture of the infant is likely to affect the results of a measurement, e.g. the position of the head and neck might affect the upper airway resistance, and because of the highly flexible chest in a newborn and load on the chest or abdomen might have an effect on lung volume and hence the elastance measurements. Most of these issues should be possible to address by standardising the procedure and training of the personnel. Another conundrum is that there are no reference data for premature infants, alas it is not normal to be born too early. We posit that the patient would become his/her own control and that the data might be best used as a tool to monitor the development of the respiratory system in preemies. It should, however, be possible to acquire reference data from full-term infants, at least for the first few days and maybe weeks of life. Undoubtedly a reliable method to assess lung health in infants would be a great achievement and has the potential to improve the outcome in preterm babies.

SUMMARY

Respiratory oscillometry has come a long way since the first steps in the mid-1950s and is now a standard procedure in numerous clinics and is widely used in clinical studies. Of course, common diseases such as asthma and COPD are well represented in the canon of oscillometry but without a doubt there are several more areas where the technology has started to make a change in how lung function is measured, be that moving into patient categories previously difficult to assess such as infants, or new approaches on how to assess disease control by using bronchodilation and challenge testing with methacholine, or expanding into diseases where the sensitivity of oscillometry might make a big change in the care of the patient as exemplified by lung transplant care. Some areas will need further research and development to move into clinical practice, thus there are exciting opportunities for both researchers and clinicians alike.

REFERENCES

1. LK Lundblad and A Robichaud, "Oscillometry of the Respiratory System. A Translational Opportunity not to be missed," Am J Physiol. – Lung Cell. Mol. Physiol., 2021 Apr.;320(6):L1038–L1056.
2. E Cho et al., "Airway Oscillometry Detects Spirometric-Silent Episodes of Acute Cellular Rejection," Am. J. Respir. Crit. Care Med., 2020 Mar.;201(12):1536–44.
3. OS Usmani, "Calling Time on Spirometry: Unlocking the Silent Zone in Acute Rejection after Lung Transplantation," Am. J. Respir. Crit. Care Med., 2020 Jun.;201(12):1468–70.

4. KC Nilsen et al., "Donor-Recipient Size Mismatch, Donor Age and Interstitial Lung Disease Are Associated with Abnormal Reactance, Resistance and Airway Closure After Bilateral Lung Transplantation," J Hear Lung Transplant. 2022 Apr.;41(4)S418–S419.

5. DR Darley et al., "Airway oscillometry parameters in baseline lung allograft dysfunction: Associations from a multicenter study," J Hear. Lung Transplant. 2023 Jan.;42(6):767–77.

6. A Fu et al., "Characterization of chronic lung allograft dysfunction phenotypes using spectral and intrabreath oscillometry," Front. Physiol., 2022 Oct.;13.

7. A Vasileva et al., "Intra-Subject Variance of Respiratory Oscillometry Reflects Graft Injury and is Associated with Acute Rejection and Chronic Lung Allograft Dysfunction (CLAD) Post Lung Transplant (LTx)," J. Hear. Lung Transplant. 2021 Apr.;40(4):S57.

8. KM Hardaker et al., "Longitudinal Utility of Peripheral Airway Function Tests in Pulmonary Graft Vs. Host Disease in Pediatric Bone Marrow Transplant Patients," Biol. Blood Marrow Transplant, 2019 Mar.;25(3): S247–S248.

9. R Louis et al., "European Respiratory Society guidelines for the diagnosis of asthma in adults," Eur. Respir. J. 2022 Sep.;60(3).

10. GG King et al., "Technical standards for respiratory oscillometry," Eur. Respir. J. 2020 Feb.;55(2):1900753.

11. H Johansson, P Wollmer, J Sundström, C Janson, and A Malinovschi, "Bronchodilator response in FOT parameters in middle-aged adults from SCAPIS: normal values and relationship to asthma and wheezing," Eur. Respir. J. 2021 Sep.;58(3).

12. E Oostveen et al., "Respiratory impedance in healthy subjects: baseline values and bronchodilator response," Eur Respir J, 2013;42:1513–23.

13. K Jetmalani et al., "Normal limits for oscillometric bronchodilator responses and relationships with clinical factors," ERJ Open Res., 2021 Sep.;7(4)00439–02021.

14. AM Cottee, LM Seccombe, C Thamrin, GG King, MJ Peters, and CS Farah, "Bronchodilator response assessed using the forced oscillation technique identifies poor asthma control with greater sensitivity than spirometry," Chest, 2020 Jan.;157(6):1435–41.

15. AM Cottee, LM Seccombe, C Thamrin, GG King, MJ Peters, and CS Farah, "Oscillometry and Asthma Control in Patients With and Without Fixed Airflow Obstruction.," J. allergy Clin. Immunol. Pract., 2022 Dec.;10(5):1260–67.e1.

16. CR Kuo, S Jabbal, and B Lipworth, "I Say IOS You Say AOS: Comparative Bias in Respiratory Impedance Measurements," Lung, 2019 Jul.;197:473–81.

17. AL Coates et al., "ERS technical standard on bronchial challenge testing: General considerations and performance of methacholine challenge tests," Eur. Respir. J., 2017 May;49:5.

18. EJ M Weersink, FJJ vd Elshout, Cv Herwaarden, and H Folgering, "Bronchial responsiveness to histamine and methacholine measured with forced expirations and with the forced oscillation technique," Respir. Med., 1995;89(5):351–56.

19. P Lebecque, S Spier, JG Lapierre, a Lamarre, R Zinman, and a L Coates, "Histamine challenge test in children using forced oscillation to measure total respiratory resistance.," Chest, 1987 Aug.;92(2):313–8.

20. H Xu, Y Gao, Y Xie, X Liang, and J Zheng, "Bronchial provocation test measured by using the forced oscillation technique to assess airway responsiveness," Allergy Asthma Proc., 2021 Sep.;42(5):E127–E134.

21. P Jara-Gutierrez, E Aguado, MG del Potro, M Fernandez-Nieto, I Mahillo, and J Sastre, "Comparison of impulse oscillometry and spirometry for detection of airway hyperresponsiveness to methacholine, mannitol, and eucapnic voluntary hyperventilation in children," Pediatr. Pulmonol., 2019 Aug.;54(8): 1162–72.

22. M Nazemiyah, K Ansarin, M Nouri-Vaskeh, T Sadegi, and A Sharifi, "Comparison of spirometry and impulse oscillometry in methacholine challenge test for the detection of airway hyperresponsiveness in adults," Tuberk. Toraks, 2021;69(1).

23. JW Yoon et al., "Early detection of airway obstruction by impulse oscillometry system in methacholine challenge testing in preschool children.," Asian Pacific J. allergy Immunol., 2018;36(3):137–44.

24. M Gazzola et al., "Airway smooth muscle tone increases airway responsiveness in healthy young adults," Am J Physiol. – Lung Cell. Mol. Physiol., 2017;312:L348–L357.

25. S Kalliola, LP Malmberg, AS Pelkonen, and MJ Mäkelä, "Aberrant small airways function relates to asthma severity in young children," Respir. Med., 2016 Feb.;111:16–20.

26. A Wong et al., "Home-based Forced Oscillation Technique Day-to-Day Variability in Pediatric Asthma," Am. J. Respir. Crit. Care Med., 2019 May.;199(9):1156–60.

27. SC Zimmermann et al., "Day-to-day variability of forced oscillatory mechanics for early detection of acute exacerbations in COPD," Eur. Respir. J., 2020 Sep.;56(3).

28. A Angelucci and A Aliverti, "Telemonitoring systems for respiratory patients: technological aspects," Pulmonology, 2020 Jul.;26(4):221–32.

29. LKA Lundblad, S Siddiqui, Y Bossé, and R Dandurand, "Applications of oscillometry in clinical research and practice," Can. J. Respir. Crit. Care Sleep Med., 2021;5(1):54–68.

30. M Schwaiblmair, W Behr, T Haeckel, B Märkl, W Foerg, and T Berghaus, "Drug Induced Interstitial Lung Disease," Open Respir Med J, 2012;6:63–74.

31. JKY Wu et al., "Correlation of respiratory oscillometry with CT image analysis in a prospective cohort of idiopathic pulmonary fibrosis," BMJ open Respir. Res., 2022 Apr.;9(1):e001163.

32. GF Nieman et al., "A Physiologically Informed Strategy to Effectively Open, Stabilize, and Protect the Acutely Injured Lung ," Frontiers in Physiology, 2020;11:227.

33. S Neelakantan et al., "Computational lung modelling in respiratory medicine," J. R. Soc. Interface, 2022;19:191.

34. FM Ducharme and GM Davis, "Measurement of respiratory resistance in the emergency department: Feasibility in young children with acute asthma," Chest, 1997;111(6):1519–25.

35. FM Ducharme, A Smyrnova, CC Lawson, and LM Miles, "Reference values for respiratory sinusoidal oscillometry in children aged 3 to 17 years," Pediatr. Pulmonol., 2022;57(9):2092–2102.

36. N Navanandan, KL Hamlington, RD Mistry, SJ Szefler, and AH Liu, "Oscillometry for acute asthma in the pediatric emergency department: A feasibility study," Ann. Allergy, Asthma Immunol., 2020;125(5): 607–609.

37. ML Vielkind et al., "Airwave oscillometry to measure lung function in children with Down syndrome," Pediatr. Res., 2021;91(7):1775–80.

38. C Calogero et al., "Respiratory impedance and bronchodilator responsiveness in healthy children aged 2–13 years," Pediatr. Pulmonol., 2013 Jul.;48(7):707–15.

39. A Dutta et al., "Impact of prenatal and postnatal household air pollution exposure on lung function of 2-year old Nigerian children by oscillometry," Sci. Total Environ., 2020 Nov.;755:143419.

40. H Knihtilä, A Kotaniemi-Syrjänen, MJ Mäkelä, J Bondestam, AS Pelkonen, and LP Malmberg, "Preschool oscillometry and lung function at adolescence in asthmatic children," Pediatr. Pulmonol., 2015 Dec.;50(12): 1205–13.

41. A Klinger et al., "Pulmonary Function Using Non-invasive Forced Oscillometry Respiratory (PUFFOR) Testing in Term Neonates," Pediatric Academic Societies Meeting, 2019. [Online]. Available: https://www.xcdsystem.com/pas/program/2019/index.cfm?pgid=157andSearchTerm=Klinger.

42. CP Travers, AP Klinger, I Aban, W Hoover, WA Carlo, and N Ambalavanan, "Non-Invasive Oscillometry to Measure Pulmonary Mechanics in Preterm Infants," Am. J. Respir. Crit. Care Med., p. rccm.202101-0226LE, May 2021.

43. E Zannin, C Rigotti, RP Neumann, RL Dellacà, S Schulzke, and ML Ventura, "Oscillatory mechanics in very preterm infants on continuous positive airway pressure support: Reference values," Pediatr. Pulmonol., 2023 Nov.;58(3):746–52.

Practice Questions and Explanations

• Thomas Vadakkan • Nishanth PS • Daksh Sharma

1. A 56-year-old chronic smoker presents with a history of prolonged cough, and expectoration during winter season for the past 5 years and presented with persisting cough with expectoration, breathlessness—5 months. FOT parameters are the following:

	$cmH_2O/L/S$ (Pre-BDR)	Post-BDR
R_5	9 (210%)	8
R_{20}	5 (180%)	5
R_{5-20}	4 (400%)	3

Most probable diagnosis:
a. COPD
b. ILD
c. Bronchial asthma
d. Upper airway obstruction
e. Retrosternal goitre

2. A 29-year-old female hospital staff who complains of episodic breathlessness, wheezing and dry cough for past 15 years. She gives history of dust allergy and sneezing. Her oscillometry readings are as follows:

	$cmH_2O/L/S$ (Pre-BDR)	$cmH_2O/L/S$ (Post-BDR)	% Change after BDR
R_5	6	4.3	50
R_{20}	3.2	3.2	Nil
R_{5-20}	2.8	1	200%

Most probable diagnosis:
a. COPD
b. CAO
c. Bronchial asthma with reversibility
d. ILD
e. Upper airway obstruction

3. A 7-year-old male boy presents with recurrent episodes of night cough for past 2 years. No history of wheezing or expectoration. His chest X-ray and spirometry unremarkable. Oscillometry values are following:

	$cmH_2O/L/S$	% Change
R_5	9	51%
R_{20}	3.9	14%
R_{5-20}	5.2	71%

Most probable clinical diagnosis:

a. COPD

b. Hypersensitivity pneumonitis

c. SAD/asthma (small airway dysfunction)

d. Upper airway obstruction

e. Bronchopulmonary dysplasia (BPD)

4. A 80-year-old reformed smoker complaining of progressive exertional dyspnea and dry cough of 2 years duration, unable to sleep last 2 weeks due to severe cough. Patient also has mild snoring and occasional knee pain. History of treatment for pneumonia 1 year back. Oscillometry parameters are following:

	$cmH_2O/L/S$	% change
R_5	3.9	1
R_{20}	3.1	2.2
R_5-R_{20}	0.97	1.9
AX	3.2	150
X_5	−2.8	−120

Most probable clinical diagnosis:

a. COPD

b. IPF

c. Inducible laryngeal obstruction/PVFM

d. Bronchial asthma

e. Retrosternal goitre

5. A 30-year-old lady, working as a school teacher, complaining of exertional dyspnea and noisy breathing. She was diagnosed from primary health centre with possible obstructive airway disease and was given inhaled corticosteroids with LABA. She has no improvement in symptoms and her chest X-ray and spirometry was unremarkable. CT chest and neck were normal. Nasal endoscopy was also normal. Oscillometry parameters are following:

	$cm/H_2O/L/S$	% change
R_5	7	75
R_{20}	8	166
R_5-R_{20}	1	0

Most probable clinical diagnosis:

a. COPD

b. IPF

c. Inducible laryngeal obstruction/PVFM

d. Bronchial asthma

e. Retrosternal goitre

6. A 40-year-old home maker recently complaining of shortness of breath, cough, palpitation, anxiety, tremor and significant weight loss more than 6 months duration. Supine position worsens her cough and dyspnea. Cardiology work up was normal except sinus tachycardia. There was no obvious swelling in throat or neck. Oscillometry parameters are following:

	$cm/H_2O/L/S$	% change
R_5	9	75
R_{20}	10	233
$R_5–R_{20}$	1	0

Most probable clinical diagnosis:

a. COPD

b. IPF

c. Inducible laryngeal obstruction/PVFM

d. Bronchial asthma

e. Retrosternal goitre

EXPLANATIONS

1. a. COPD

In COPD there will be both peripheral and central airway obstruction.

In combined airway obstruction R_5, R_{20}, $R_{5–20}$, A_x, F_{res} will be increased, X_5 will be more negative.

The mean values of R_5, $R_{5–20}$, A_x, X_5 and F_{res} progressively worsened as GOLD severity increased. In contrast R_{20} values were similar at all GOLD stages.

The A_x ≥8.66 cmH_2O/L has ability for diagnosing COPD. The diagnostic ability of IOS parameters for detection of COPD was high when compared between COPD with low % predicted of FEV_1 and chronic smokers. In chronic obstructive pulmonary disease (COPD), a decrease in X_5 suggests dynamic hyperinflation. Difference in inspiratory reactance (XI) and expiratory reactance (XE) correlate with COPD severity.

These findings indicate that IOS is an useful tool for diagnosis of COPD especially in the subjects who cannot perform spirometry.

2. c. BA with reversibility

In pure small airway obstruction/small airway dysfunction (SAD) as in bronchial asthma R_5 and $R_{5–20}$ will be increased

Parameters to suggest bronchodilator reversibility in lung oscillometry are reduction in R_5 >40%, X_5 >50%, A_x >80%.

3. c. BA with normal spirometry/SAD

Here in this question, R_5 and $R_{5–20}$ are increased, with only a minimal elevation R_{20}. Lung oscillometry is better in determining early small airway dysfunction (SAD) particularly in pediatric population in whom spirometry is unremarkable or who are unable to perform the spirometry correctly, often leading to delayed diagnosis.

Control of asthma is said to be poor if associated with increased $R_{5–20}$, X_5, A_x, even in the background of normal spirometry.

4. b. Interstitial lung disease/IPF

Patient's age of 80 years, smoking history, and progressive nature of dyspnea and dry cough points towards interstitial lung disease most probably IPF. In restrictive lung diseases, R_5, R_{20}, R_{5-20} will be normal, X_5 will be more negative and A_x, F_{res} will be increased.

5. c. PVFM/inducible laryngeal obstruction

Here in this question R_5 increased, R_5–R_{20} normal and R_{20} markedly increased. Since nasal endoscopy, CT neck and CT chest are normal, this isolates the pathology to vocal cord. Since the subject is a school teacher and on a background of poor voice hygiene, it is a case of paroxysmal vocal fold motion disorder (PVFMD) which is recently renamed as inducible laryngeal obstruction.

6. e. Central airway obstruction

This is a case of retrosternal goitre with tracheal compression causing symptoms of proximal/central airway obstruction.

In central airway obstruction, Both R_5 and R_{20} will rise equally (with normal R_{5-20}), which will be frequency independent.

Though the patient was not having any obvious neck swelling, symptoms were due to retrosternal goitre compressing the trachea and her hyperthyroid status.

REFERENCE VALUES

R_5	–	4
R_{20}	–	3
R_{5-20}	–	1
X_5	–	-1
A_x	–	4